TRIMMING YOUR WAISTLINE

TRIMMING YOUR WAISTLINE
Ten Steps to Better Health and Fitness

R. MATHENY, PHD, RDN

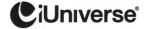

TRIMMING YOUR WAISTLINE
TEN STEPS TO BETTER HEALTH AND FITNESS

iUniverse books may be ordered through booksellers or by contacting:

iUniverse
1663 Liberty Drive
Bloomington, IN 47403
www.iuniverse.com
1-800-Authors (1-800-288-4677)

ISBN: 978-1-5320-6242-1 (sc)
ISBN: 978-1-5320-6241-4 (e)

Library of Congress Control Number: 2018913717

Print information available on the last page.

iUniverse rev. date: 02/13/2019

In memory of my parents for their invaluable guidance and unconditional love throughout the years. Also, in memory of my dear friend Ruth Flygare, who supported the writing of my two books. She was a quiet presence but made a huge impact on those she touched. Most of all, a thank-you to our Lord God and His Son for all that is meaningful in life.

Contents

Preface

When I was in grade school, I had the idea that I would like to teach. My career in public health has given me opportunity to do that. Based on my experiences with working with families that have infants, toddlers, and preschoolers and my training in child development, I wrote my first book, *A Healthy Weight: The Best Birthday Gift for Your Child*, which provides nutrition information to prevent or correct obesity in infants to teens.

I was a chubby teen. Over the years, I have worked hard to eat in a healthy way to control my weight and continue to do so. However, I have never forgotten how sensitive people's feelings can be concerning appearance and weight. Presently, there are millions of men and women in our country who are overweight or obese. For this reason, I want to share with them who are dieting to identify and correct the practices that have caused their weight problems and share with them how to lose these extra pounds wisely. Last, as a public health nutritionist, I enjoyed counseling expectant mothers concerning eating healthily and following weight-gain recommendations so they could have healthy babies. The advice in this book can help mothers who gained weight during pregnancy and who desire to lose the unwanted pounds.

Acknowledgments

Acknowledgment and warm thanks to my sister, Mary, and my brother, Bill, and his family for their continued support. Also, great appreciation to Debra Scurry and Brenda Eads for their advice and technical assistance with the writing of this book, Sue Carson for its artwork, and the editorial staff of iUniverse for their valuable recommendations. Sincere appreciation to Chris Cutler, MS, RD, experienced in clinical dietetics, for reviewing the book's content and to Saprina Matheny, MSW, licensed independent social worker for review of chapters 3 and 4. Also warm thanks to the staff of my local library, Robert Pierson, and his assistants, Mary Becker and Michelle Marvin, for helping me acquire the professional resources required for the writing of this book.

Introduction: A Healthy Way to a Healthy Weight

There are many popular diets that offer quick fixes and weight-loss supplements that are thought to have magical powers that are very appealing to dieters because they promise instant weight loss. Because the rapid weight reduction is due mainly to the loss of body water, not fat, dieters quickly regain the weight that has been lost once they stop the diet. Rapid weight loss can also cause medical problems. In addition, if these diets and supplements have such magical powers, why are there millions of American men and women who remain overweight and obese and more becoming so?

The Approach to This Book

An old adage I learned in my public health training is "Give a man a fish, he will eat for a day. Teach a man how to fish, he will eat for a lifetime." When you visit bookstores online, you will discover that there are many, many books that have different approaches to weight loss. In addition, there are numerous weight-reduction programs that offer a diet plan and meals to support them. However, because many of the weight-loss plans have features that lose their appeal and become too expensive over time, they are discontinued. Why? These weight-loss plans and weight-reduction programs do not target the question that gets to the root of the problem—what are the problems that have caused you to gain the weight in the first place?

The purpose of this book is to provide practical advice to prevent or correct weight problems in men and women that are reducing their quality of life. In addition, this information could be helpful to health professionals in the area of weight management and the paraprofessionals who assist them. The approach in this book offers you and other dieters a hands-on, step-by-step experience that answers not only what problems have caused you to gain the extra pounds but also how to correct them.

Why hands-on? It is important that you are in charge. You will be asked to make important decisions that will help your weight-loss and weight-maintenance efforts be successful. You will be asked to

- identify the unhealthy practices that have caused you to gain weight;

- select among a number of practical solutions to correct these problems;

- select weight-loss and weight-maintenance plans and develop a physical activity plan that best match your personal needs and preferences;

- keep monitoring records that will track your dietary intake, weight you have lost, and physical activities you have done;

- make commitments (goals) that summarize your willingness to adopt practical solutions to correct unhealthy practices; and

- follow your weight-loss, weight-maintenance, and physical-activity plans to reduce your weight and to maintain the new one.

Your Lifelong Journey to Better Health and Fitness

While you are on this journey to *better health* and *fitness*, think about the colors of a traffic light

- Green: Go get them!

- Yellow: Don't waver along the way!

- Red: Stop only when you obtain your goals!

You will be asked to take ten steps. These are the chapter titles that reflect the book's in-depth and personalized approach to weight management:

- Chapter 1: Taking a Look at Your Weight: The first step is to evaluate your weight (normal weight, overweight, or obese).

- Chapter 2: Taking a Look at Your Health: The second step is to evaluate your health.

- Chapter 3: Preparing Yourself Mentally for the Task of Losing Weight: The third step is to adopt positive thoughts about yourself and your body.

- Chapter 4: Stress Management: The fourth step is to reduce your level of stress.

- Chapter 5: Basic Nutrition Facts: The fifth step is to become acquainted with important nutrition information.

- Chapter 6: Determining What Is Right or Wrong with Your Dietary Intake: The sixth step is to take a closer look at the quality of your dietary intake.

- Chapter 7: Determining What Is Right or Wrong with Your Eating Practices: The seventh step is to carefully examine your eating practices.

- Chapter 8: Selecting a Weight-Loss Plan and Setting Dietary Goals: The eighth step is to start reducing your weight.

- Chapter 9: Planning Your Physical Fitness Program: The ninth step is to improve your physical fitness.

- Chapter 10: Weight Maintenance: The tenth step is to tally your improvements and think about weight maintenance.

Balance is the key to success. The concept of balance is emphasized throughout the chapters.

Because of the interrelated nature of the chapters, it is very important that you do not skip chapters. Relevant internet resources appear throughout the chapters. If you do not use the computer or do not have access to one, check with your local librarian to inquire about available computer services or the interlibrary loan system.

Take charge, for you are in the driver's seat. The ten steps can serve as goals. These goals can act as a road map, guiding you in the right direction. The monitoring forms you keep will act as a compass, keeping you on track. The *evaluations* you complete will be the road signs that record and reward your progress to a healthier lifestyle.

This book can provide you the opportunity to lose weight and the means of rewarding your progress. You will have to supply the enthusiasm to learn and a strong motivation to do the work. Most importantly, have faith in yourself, and be confident that you will succeed in achieving your weight-loss and weight-maintenance goals. Ask family members, friends, and coworkers to support or join you in these efforts.

When I was conducting weight-reduction classes, one of my larger participants came up to me after class and asked if she could come in to the health department and weigh herself weekly. She faithfully did so. The last time I saw her, because I was leaving to acquire my graduate degree, she had lost quite a bit of weight and happily commented, "I can get into some of my clothes that I haven't worn for years." I was pleased for her as well. Although I will not be right there with you in your efforts to lose weight, I will be on the sidelines rooting you on all the way. Good luck!

CHAPTER
1

Taking a Look at Your Weight

Obesity in our country is reaching alarming levels and is becoming a serious health problem. Why is this happening? Many Americans are consuming too many calories because of unhealthy eating practices (calories in). At the same time, they are using too few calories because of limited physical activity (calories out).

Our bodies work hard to maintain a balance so that when our calories in equal our calories out, we maintain our weight. In contrast, when our calories in are higher than our calories out, unwanted pounds accumulate, and we gain excess weight. This excess weight can increase our risk for disease. The first step on your road to better health and fitness is to improve your weight to reduce your risk for disease.

Body Mass Index

You most likely have heard the term *body mass index* on news reports concerning health. Body mass index (BMI) uses your height and weight. Nutrition and medical professionals describe BMI as a measure of total body fat.[1]

How can I determine my body mass index? See the table of BMI values that follows.[2] These values are for adult men and non-pregnant women. Follow the top row of heights until you find your height. Next, look down the row of BMI values until you find the BMI that is in line with your weight on the left. For example, for a height of five feet, five inches and a weight of 170 pounds, the BMI is 28. If your weight is not on the table and is half or more between two values, select the higher weight. For example if your weight is 168 pounds, select 170. Follow these steps to obtain your height and weight:

1. It is recommended that you determine your height (to the nearest inch) at your physician's office on a standardized scale after removing your shoes and socks.

2. It is recommended that you weigh yourself in the morning around the same time every day before eating breakfast and wearing lightweight undergarments or a robe, without any type of footwear. Be sure when you purchase a scale that you check its weighing capacity. Most scales have a weighing capacity between 300 and 350 pounds. Weighing can reveal the problem but also track positive changes.

Table of BMI Values

How To Determine BMI

Height (Feet and Inches)

Weight (Pounds)	5'0"	5'1"	5'2"	5'3"	5'4"	5'5"	5'6"	5'7"	5'8"	5'9"	5'10"	5'11"	6'0"	6'1"	6'2"	6'3"	6'4"
100	20	19	18	18	17	17	16	16	15	15	14	14	14	13	13	12	12
105	21	20	19	19	18	17	17	16	16	16	15	15	14	14	13	13	13
110	21	21	20	19	19	18	18	17	17	16	16	15	15	15	14	14	13
115	22	22	21	20	20	19	19	18	17	17	17	16	16	15	15	14	14
120	23	23	22	21	21	20	19	19	18	18	17	17	16	16	15	15	15
125	24	24	23	22	21	21	20	20	19	18	18	17	17	16	16	16	15
130	25	25	24	23	22	22	21	20	20	19	19	18	18	17	17	16	16
135	26	26	25	24	23	22	22	21	21	20	19	19	18	18	17	17	16
140	27	26	26	25	24	23	23	22	21	21	20	20	19	18	18	17	17
145	28	27	27	26	25	24	23	23	22	21	21	20	20	19	19	18	18
150	29	28	27	27	26	25	24	23	23	22	22	21	20	20	19	19	18
155	30	29	28	27	27	26	25	24	24	23	22	22	21	20	20	19	19
160	31	30	29	28	27	27	26	25	24	24	23	22	22	21	21	20	19
165	32	31	30	29	28	27	27	26	25	24	24	23	22	22	21	21	20
170	33	32	31	30	29	28	27	27	26	25	24	24	23	22	22	21	21
175	34	33	32	31	30	29	28	27	27	26	25	24	24	23	22	22	21
180	35	34	33	32	31	30	29	28	27	27	26	25	24	24	23	22	22
185	36	35	34	33	32	31	30	29	28	27	27	26	25	24	24	23	23
190	37	36	35	34	33	32	31	30	29	28	27	26	26	25	24	24	23
195	38	37	36	35	33	32	31	31	30	29	28	27	26	26	25	24	24
200	39	38	37	35	34	33	32	31	30	30	29	28	27	26	26	25	24
205	40	39	37	36	35	34	33	32	31	30	29	29	28	27	26	26	25
210	41	40	38	37	36	35	34	33	32	31	30	29	28	28	27	26	26
215	42	41	39	38	37	36	35	34	33	32	31	30	29	28	28	27	26
220	43	42	40	39	38	37	36	34	33	32	32	31	30	29	28	27	27
225	44	43	41	40	39	37	36	35	34	33	32	31	31	30	29	28	27
230	45	43	42	41	39	38	37	36	35	34	33	32	31	30	30	29	28
235	46	44	43	42	40	39	38	37	36	35	34	33	32	31	30	29	29
240	47	45	44	43	41	40	39	38	36	35	34	33	33	32	31	30	29
245	48	46	45	43	42	41	40	38	37	36	35	34	33	32	31	31	30
250	49	47	46	44	43	42	40	39	38	37	36	35	34	33	32	31	30

For individuals not covered by this table, calculate BMI by converting pounds to kilograms (1 pound = 0.45 kilograms) and inches to meters (1 inch = .0254 meters).
The equation for BMI is weight (in kilograms) divided by height (in meters) squared [kg/m^2].
Source: *Shape Up America!*, 6707 Democracy Blvd., Suite 107, Bethesda, MD 20817

How To Determine BMI

Height (Feet and Inches)

Weight (Pounds)	5'0"	5'1"	5'2"	5'3"	5'4"	5'5"	5'6"	5'7"	5'8"	5'9"	5'10"	5'11"	6'0"	6'1"	6'2"	6'3"	6'4"
255	50	48	47	45	44	42	41	40	39	38	37	36	35	34	33	32	31
260	51	49	48	46	45	43	42	41	40	38	37	36	35	34	33	32	32
265	52	50	48	47	45	44	43	42	40	39	38	37	36	35	34	33	32
270	53	51	49	48	46	45	44	42	41	40	39	38	37	36	35	34	33
275	54	52	50	49	47	46	44	43	42	41	39	38	37	36	35	34	33
280	55	53	51	50	48	47	45	44	43	41	40	39	38	37	36	35	34
285	56	54	52	50	49	47	46	45	43	42	41	40	39	38	37	36	35
290	57	55	53	51	50	48	47	45	44	43	42	40	39	38	37	36	35
295	58	56	54	52	51	49	48	46	45	44	42	41	40	39	38	37	36
300	59	57	55	53	51	50	48	47	46	44	43	42	41	40	39	37	37
305	60	58	56	54	52	51	49	48	46	45	44	43	41	40	39	38	37
310	61	59	57	55	53	52	50	49	47	46	44	43	42	41	40	39	38
315	62	60	58	56	54	52	51	49	48	47	45	44	43	42	40	39	38
320	62	60	59	57	55	53	52	50	49	47	46	45	43	42	41	40	39
325	63	61	59	58	56	54	52	51	49	48	47	45	44	43	42	41	40
330	64	62	60	58	57	55	53	52	50	49	47	46	45	44	42	41	40
335	65	63	61	59	58	56	54	52	51	49	48	47	45	44	43	42	41
340	66	64	62	60	58	57	55	53	52	50	49	47	46	45	44	42	41
345	67	65	63	61	59	57	56	54	52	51	50	48	47	46	44	43	42
350	68	66	64	62	60	58	56	55	53	52	50	49	47	46	45	44	43
355	69	67	65	63	61	59	57	56	54	52	51	50	48	47	46	44	43
360	70	68	66	64	62	60	58	56	55	53	52	50	49	47	46	45	44
365	71	69	67	65	63	61	59	57	55	54	52	51	50	48	47	46	44
370	72	70	68	66	64	62	60	58	56	55	53	52	50	49	48	46	45
375	73	71	69	66	64	62	61	59	57	55	54	52	51	49	48	47	46
380	74	72	70	67	65	63	61	60	58	56	55	53	52	50	49	47	46
385	75	73	70	68	66	64	62	60	59	57	55	54	52	51	49	48	47
390	76	74	71	69	67	65	63	61	59	58	56	54	53	51	50	49	47
395	77	75	72	70	68	66	64	62	60	58	57	55	54	52	51	49	48
400	78	76	73	71	69	67	65	63	61	59	57	56	54	53	51	50	49

For individuals not covered by this table, calculate BMI by converting pounds to kilograms (1 pound = 0.45 kilograms) and inches to meters (1 inch = .0254 meters). The equation for BMI is weight (in kilograms) divided by height (in meters) squared [kg/m^2].

Source: *Shape Up America!*, 6707 Democracy Blvd., Suite 107, Bethesda, MD 20817

How is your BMI related to your weight status? BMI can identify your weight status [1]

- normal weight: 18.5 to 24.9

- overweight: 25.0 to 29.9

- obesity class I: 30 to 34.9

- obesity class II: 35 to 39.9

- extreme obesity: 40 or more

I would recommend the following:

- If you do not have a weight problem, determine your BMI yearly.

- If you have lost weight and are maintaining it, determine your BMI every six months.

- If you are losing weight, determine your BMI every three months.

- For the first two cases, if you notice that you are gradually gaining weight, determine your BMI and take measures to halt it.

How does your BMI relate to your risk for disease? Of medical concern is that as your BMI increases, so does your risk for disease.

Focus on the Positive

For you dieters who are overweight or obese, you may be a bit discouraged at this point, and the task of losing weight may be daunting. However, to reduce these feelings, let us take a closer look at the table of BMI values:

- In many cases, a weight loss of five pounds can result in a change of one BMI value.

- Thus, it must be emphasized here that in some cases, a weight loss of twenty-five pounds can change a person's weight status by five BMI values.

- This means that if you are overweight, you could reduce this to a normal weight status, and if you are obese and have a BMI value between 30 to 34, you could reduce your weight status to overweight.

- For those with BMI values above 35, reducing your weight by five BMI values is beneficial as well.

- By reducing your BMI by five values, you make a significant impact on your risk for disease.

- Check the BMI table to see how many BMI value changes there would be if you lost twenty-five or fifty pounds.

Waist Circumference

Waist circumference is excess abdominal fat.[1] Basically, this is fat within the waistline area. I would recommend that you do the following:

1. If you do not have a weight problem, determine your waist circumference yearly.

2. If you have lost weight and are maintaining it, determine your waist circumference every six months.

3. If you are gaining weight, determine your waist circumference every three months.

4. For the first two cases, if you notice that you are gradually gaining weight, determine your waist circumference and take measures to halt it.

How can I determine my waist circumference? Taking waist circumference measurements is mainly done in research studies. However, there is a practical way you can obtain your measurements. For men, the waistbands of pants are already given in inches. For women, pants are marketed by petite, regular, and extra-large sizes. I would recommend that you purchase a nonstretchable tape measure. Attach this tape measure by paper clips or safety pins around the waistband to determine the band size in inches.

For both men and women, the pants used to obtain waist circumference should not have stretchable waistbands.

Why is it important that I know my waist circumference? Similar to BMI, waist circumference can identify your level of risk for disease. Men who have waist circumference greater than forty inches and women who have waist circumference greater than thirty-five inches are at higher risk for diabetes, dyslipidemia, hypertension, and cardiovascular disease.[1] Dieters who have circumferences of forty or thirty-five inches or less are at a lower risk for such diseases.

I know that some of you who have weight problems prefer not having your picture taken. However, I would recommend that you have one of your supporters take a photo of you at the beginning and then again at three months and six months into your weight-loss efforts. Visually witnessing the removal of those unwanted pounds by these three snapshots in time can give you a big boost in your self-confidence and in your health as well.

ENDNOTES

1 National Institutes of Health, National Heart, Lung, and Blood Institute, U.S. Department of Health and Human Services, and North American Associates for the Study of Obesity. *The Practical Guide Identification, Evaluation, and Treatment of Overweight and Obesity in Adults.* Bethesda, MD: NIH Publication Number 02-4084, 2002

2 *Guidance for Treatment of Adult Obesity.* Bethesda, MD: Shape Up America and American Obesity Association, 1996.

CHAPTER 2

Taking a Look at Your Health

If you glance through this chapter, you will notice a number of medical terms. You most likely have heard some of these terms while visiting your physician's office or listening to news reports on health issues. The information in this chapter is not to persuade you to lose weight as a result of scare tactics, such as "reduce your weight or else …" Its purpose is to answer the question "Why does excess weight cause disease?"

Recall that when our calories in are higher than our calories out, excess weight is gained. I think of excess weight as a biological spark plug that sets into motion a number of events in the body that lead to disease. These events will become clearer in this chapter. In addition, a fictitious patient's medical experience will be used as a case study to illustrate how excess weight and its consequences are related to present-day diagnosis and treatment. The second step on your road to better health and fitness is to become an informed patient to improve your health.

Excess Weight as a Biological Spark Plug

Excess weight acts as a biological spark plug that sets into motion a number of events in the body that lead to disease. In light of this, those unwanted pounds are definitely *unhealthy* ones.

Event 1

Excess weight due to unhealthy eating and limited physical activity produces a number of unhealthy changes in our bodies, such as abnormal changes in the blood pressure and blood clotting systems and in the use of glucose, cholesterol, and fat.

Event 2

These unhealthy changes trigger a number of *metabolic abnormalities* which could include:[1]

- increased blood pressure

- increased blood glucose levels

- increased blood LDL-cholesterol (LDL-c)

- decreased blood HDL-cholesterol (HDL-c)

- increased triglyceride (fat) levels

- increased blood clotting

HDL-c is beneficial to health while LDL-c is harmful. Undoubtedly, there are more *metabolic abnormalities*, but I focus on these six because they are the most often used in medical diagnosis. Realize that as each of these *metabolic abnormalities* become more abnormal in value and as more abnormalities become present in your medical picture, your risk for disease will be greater.

Event 3

Unfortunately, these *metabolic abnormalities* silently damage vital organs and blood vessels until they no longer function properly, contributing to type 2 diabetes, heart disease, high blood pressure, and stroke.[1]

Treatment Approaches

The wise advice of Benjamin Franklin is, an ounce of prevention is worth a pound of cure remains more meaningful today in light of the magnitude of the obesity problem and the severity of its diseases. As a public health nutritionist, I am concerned about the human cost of obesity. The chronic diseases that could cause death and the weight-related problems that are painful and debilitating (loss of physical function, such as orthopedic problems) are emotionally devastating and physically draining. Top these off with the emotional scars that are time after time opened by society's negativity and critical comments by others targeted at one's weight, whether one is overweight or obese. To sum up, the price tag attached to obesity is a compromised health and quality of life, both physically and emotionally, not only for the person but for his or her loved ones as well. There are many medical and nutrition professionals who want to help. All we ask when you come to us is to have an open mind and to listen to our recommendations. Take them to heart so you will follow them, and stick with them so they will become lifelong practices.

Medical Diagnosis

Referring to event 2, whether one, a few, or all of the *metabolic abnormali*ties are present will depend on (1) the amount of excess weight determined by your BMI and your waist circumference and (2) your genetic makeup determined by your family history of genetic predispositions to the chronic diseases (obesity, heart disease, high blood pressure, stroke, and type 2 diabetes).

How do these relate to medical diagnosis and treatment? Consider the following:

1. When your blood pressure is taken at your physician's office, it will be evaluated as normal, borderline high, or abnormally high.

2. When your blood is taken and analyzed for glucose, LDL-c, triglycerides, blood clotting, and HDL-c levels, the laboratory results will be evaluated as normal, borderline high, low, or abnormally high in the case of the first four and low for HDL-c levels.

3. Your doctor will evaluate all of the above as normal, borderline, or abnormal, along with any weight-related problems identified upon your physical exam, family history of disease, medical history, and present eating and physical activity practices. This will help your physician to decide the dosage of medication that best matches your medical picture.

Supportive Medications

Individuals who are taking medications prescribed for abnormal blood pressure, glucose, cholesterol, triglycerides, and blood clotting may need to take additional steps to decrease their risk for disease. Excess weight is not only a medical problem, but a nutritional one as well. Medications such as those prescribed for abnormal blood pressure, glucose, cholesterol, triglycerides, and blood clotting can only control their respective *metabolic abnormalities*, but they cannot correct the primary reason for the problem which is excess weight caused by unhealthy eating habits and physical inactivity. Accordingly, such medications should be viewed as playing a supportive role in therapy. In other words, total reliance on medication for treatment should be avoided.

It is important to know that specific drugs within the above medicine categories may cause weight gain. If you suspect that one of these drugs is causing weight gain, ask your local pharmacist if this is true and if there is an alternative that does not. If so, ask your physician if he or she will approve this alternative. In many cases, supportive medications may be adjusted (dosage lowered) or discontinued in response to the improved medical profile resulting from weight loss and physical activity.

Weight-Loss Medications and Supplements

It is strongly advised that you do not purchase weight-loss medications or supplements through the internet or television. Prescribed weight-loss medications need to be approved by and under the supervision of your physician. He or she can determine dosage level, duration, and effectiveness so adverse side effects can be avoided.

Weight-loss medications are most effective when used in conjunction with a nutritionally balanced weight-loss or weight-maintenance plan and increased physical activity. However, quite often once the weight-loss medication (or supplement) is discontinued, weight is regained. These medications are not magic and are not meant to be used indefinitely.

I would not recommend weight-loss supplements. Why? The safety, content, and effectiveness of these products are not guaranteed, because they can be marketed without the approval of the Federal Drug Administration (FDA).

Weight-loss supplements may contain a stimulant, such as tea, that can increase blood pressure. This could be harmful in dieters who already have an existing blood pressure problem. Such supplements may be costly to not only your health but also your pocketbook because they are expensive.

Nutrition Recommendations

Excess weight is treatable. The best therapy is under your control. Weight reduction and increased physical activity can lessen or correct not only the health complications but also the emotional stress associated with the weight-related diseases.

Recall that excess weight is caused by unhealthy eating habits and limited physical activity. Presently, Americans are eating more meals and snacks outside of the home, especially fast food–type meals and snacks, which are high in calories, cholesterol, fat, and salt. They are also eating too many foods that are high in fat and sugar or salt, such as desserts, pastries, french fries, chips, and sweetened beverages, such as soft drinks and sweetened tea.

The weight-loss plans in this book provide a healthy balance of nutrients and can assist you with weight reduction. The diets focus on fat-free or lower-fat dairy products; lean meats; fruits and vegetables; whole-grain breads, cereals, and pastas; and monounsaturated and omega-3 fats. It is also recommended that you minimize your intake of foods high in fat and sugar or salt, sweetened beverages, and meals and snacks taken outside of the home.

The Role of Genetics

Excess weight can add to the *metabolic abnormalities* seen in patients with a genetic predisposition to disease, such as type 2 diabetes, heart disease, high blood pressure, and stroke. Reduction in weight can have a beneficial effect, but for such dieters, because of the severity of the disease, continued drug treatment may be required.

The Unseen Metabolic Pirate

Recall that excess weight produces *metabolic abnormalities* that can silently damage vital blood vessels and organs. The best time is now to apply the medical and nutritional recommendations described previously.

Because of individual differences in genetic makeup, some dieters may be unable to reach the BMI normal weight range. In this case, if you have one or more *metabolic abnormalities*, it would be best to adopt the recommended healthy eating practices and increase your physical activity so your blood pressure, glucose, LDL-c and HDL-c, and triglyceride levels can be corrected. This recommendation applies to other dieters as well. *Consider a mixture of metabolic abnormalities as a metabolic pirate.* Don't let the metabolic pirate include your health and quality of life as part of *his* treasure.

I want to emphasize here that correcting excess weight is under your control—that is, it can be corrected. In the following chapters, I have identified the unhealthy practices that contribute to excess weight and practical recommendations to correct them. Remember you are in charge. You can identify the unhealthy practices that have caused your weight problem and follow the recommendations to correct them so you can improve your health and achieve the quality of life you deserve.

Workbook of My Progress

Often individuals are reluctant to undergo a physical examination and to have blood drawn for laboratory analyses. However, to get the full advantage of the weight-loss program set forth by this book, I would strongly recommend that you keep a workbook, by using either a spiral notebook or a computer. Think positive! Name this book "Workbook of My Progress." In this workbook, you will be asked to write down the results requested by the different chapters. For example, in chapter 1, write down the results based on information about your BMI and waist circumference at the beginning and then again at three months and at six months into your weight-loss efforts.

In chapter 2, write down your blood pressure readings and whether they are normal, borderline high, or abnormal at the beginning, at three months, and at six months. I suggest writing down your blood pressure findings at each visit. Also, write down the results of the laboratory analyses of your blood levels of glucose, LDL-c, HDL-c, and triglycerides and whether they are normal, borderline, or abnormal at the beginning and at six months. If it is possible for you and your physician, blood results at three months would be recommended if the initial results of a specific blood constituent was borderline or abnormal. In addition, if you are taking a supportive medication, such as one to reduce glucose or blood pressure, reevaluation of this specific constituent may need to be done more often. Remember that as weight is lost, the dosage of a medication may be reduced or discontinued. Check with your physician. Last, write down the medications prescribed at the beginning, three months, and six months.

Practical pointers include the following:

- Call to make appointments with your physician, and explain that you are trying to reduce your weight and would like to have your blood pressure taken and laboratory analysis of your blood.

- Request early-morning appointments (before consuming breakfast) so that the laboratory results will be done on the fasting levels of blood constituents.

- Be sure to ask your physician to analyze for blood glucose and order a full lipid panel, which will include the levels of LDL-c, HDL-c, and triglycerides.

- Ask your physician to explain the results of your blood pressure readings and laboratory tests in terms of whether they are within the normal range, borderline abnormal, or abnormal. Request a copy of the laboratory results.

Reducing your BMI and waist circumference and improving your blood pressure and the key levels of blood constituents can be very rewarding and a strong encouragement to continue your weight-loss efforts. By tracking your medical information and your medications, you can determine how effective your weight-loss efforts are in terms of improving your medical parameters and reducing your intake of associated medications. Instead of quick-fix diets, the positive changes emphasize the benefits that can be achieved through a carefully planned weight-reduction program. To illustrate the importance of this workbook, a patient's case study is provided below.

If you are overweight and do not have a blood pressure problem or any of the blood-related risk factors, and if you wish to maintain your weight as this time, it is highly advised that you read the remaining chapters as well. These chapters are relevant not only to weight reduction but also to the prevention of weight gain.

Gather Your Supportive Troops

Approach family members, relatives, friends, and coworkers to be part of your support team or as supportive partners. Try to meet every two weeks or at a time interval preferred to discuss the recommendations of this book and what you have written in your workbooks, share ideas, and exchange experiences.

A Patient's Medical Experience

I have created a medical experience for this patient to show you how the medical concepts and diagnosis and the medical and nutrition recommendations in these last two chapters came together to provide her with a positive medical experience that improved not only her health but her emotional well-being as well. This patient and the information about people in the following chapters have also been created by the author.

This patient is a twenty-seven-year-old secretary for a local law firm. As a result, her lifestyle is basically sedentary. She does not smoke or drink alcoholic beverages. This patient is a single parent, raising a six-year-old daughter. Her husband died last year of brain cancer. Because of her weight, this sorrow, and the stress of making a living for her and her daughter, she has been experiencing bouts of depression. Jane's mother, two friends, and a coworker wanted to be part of her support team because they wanted to lose weight as well.

At the beginning of her weight-reduction program, her height was five feet, five inches, and her weight was 168 pounds. Based on her height and weight, her baseline BMI value was 28, and her BMI classification was overweight. Also, her waist circumference was thirty-six inches (a high-risk circumference).

At her first appointment, from her medical history and examination, this patient had no serious diseases, but gastric reflux disease and depression were identified. Her physician prescribed a total daily dosage of 20 mg of an antidepression medication and 300 mg of a medication to reduce her reflux problem. She confided to her physician that during her bouts of depression, she often overate.

- Her blood pressure was high at 142/84 mm Hg.

- Her LDL cholesterol level was borderline at 141 mg/dL.

- It was determined that the high blood pressure and borderline cholesterol were due in part to her weight, waist circumference, physical inactivity, and stress and in part her family history of premature heart disease. Her laboratory results (mg/dL) were within the normal ranges—that is, less than 100 or 5.7 percent A1c for glucose, less than 150 for triglycerides, and 50 or more for HDL-c.

A registered dietitian gave her the following advice:

- She would follow a low-calorie weight-loss plan that would enable her to lose about twenty-five pounds over a six-month period.

- This plan included lower-fat dairy products, lean meats, fruits and vegetables, whole-grain products, and an emphasis on monounsaturated and omega-3 fats.

- Because of her high blood pressure, she was advised to watch her use of salt and reduce her intake of salty foods. She wanted to gradually increase her daily activity level from sedentary to briskly walking with her daughter sixty minutes for three days and then five days a week. She and her daughter volunteered to clean their church after services on Sunday (sixty minutes). In addition, she enrolled in a square-dancing class (sixty minutes) once a week at a local community college. This increased exercise would not only help her to reduce her weight, but it could also improve her cardio-respiratory health, reduce stress and depression, and build self-esteem.

To reduce her blood pressure and cholesterol levels, she decided to reduce her weight, following a low-fat, low-sodium diet, and to improve her physical fitness rather than taking medication. Her physician also believed that a twenty-five-pound weight loss and improved physical activity would reduce her blood pressure and improve her cholesterol levels. Because of her concern over the above medical findings, Jane was very serious about reducing her weight and increasing her physical activity, so that no medication to promote weight loss was recommended. However, her doctor prescribed medications for reflux disease and depression. At three months, these decisions were reassessed.

At three months she had lost twelve pounds. Although her weight status remained as overweight, her BMI value was reduced from twenty-eight to twenty-six. Her waist circumference was reduced from thirty-six to thirty-four inches (a waist circumference of low risk).

Note that a modest weight loss of twelve pounds and a reduction in waist circumference by two inches can positively affect blood pressure and cholesterol levels.

- Her baseline blood pressure was reduced from 142/84 (high) to 129/79 mm Hg (borderline).

- Her LDL cholesterol level remained borderline but was reduced from 141 to 122 mg/dL.

- Her glucose, triglyceride, and HDL-c levels remained within normal ranges.

She also increased her exercise level of briskly walking to five days weekly and continued to clean her church and attend a dance class, which positively influenced these parameters. In light of these positive changes, she was advised to continue the same weight-reduction plan. Because she was still having trouble with reflux disease and depression, the same medications and their total daily dosages were recommended.

At six months, she had lost twenty-two pounds. As a result, her BMI value became twenty-four, placing her in the normal weight range. Her waist circumference was reduced by two inches from thirty-four to thirty-two inches (low risk).

She continued her brisk walking, five days weekly, and continued cleaning the church and attending her dance class. Her further weight loss, reduced waist circumference, and continued physical activity resulted in the following:

- Her blood pressure was reduced from 129/79 (borderline) to 119/76 mm Hg (normal).

- Her LDL cholesterol was reduced from 122 (borderline) to 99 mg/ dL (normal).

- Her glucose, triglyceride, and HDL-c levels remained within normal ranges.

Because of her family history of heart disease, her physician stressed the importance of continuing a diet lower in fat and salt and high in fiber, and maintaining her present weight and improved level of physical activity. Over the six months, with more regular meals, smaller portion sizes, and careful selections of food, her episodes of gastric reflux became less frequent. Because of her positive changes in weight, exercise, and health status, she experienced fewer periods of depression.

In addition, she started dating a faculty member of the college where she was taking dance lessons. Consequently, her medications were reduced from *total daily dosages* of 20 to 10 mg for depression and from 300 to 150 mg for the reflux problem. At this time she is more physically fit, and her medical picture has improved because her laboratory results were all within healthy ranges. She, however, would like to lose ten or fifteen more pounds but after her six-month maintenance period. Like this patient, you can discuss the results of your physical with your doctor to open a window to your health.

Patient with her physician

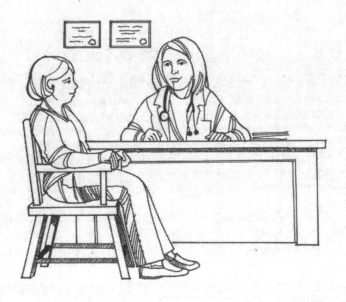

ENDNOTE

1   National Institutes of Health, National Heart, Lung, and Blood Institute, U.S. Department of Health and Human Services, and North American Associates for the Study of Obesity. *The Practical Guide Identification, Evaluation, and Treatment of Overweight and Obesity in Adults.* Bethesda, MD: NIH Publication Number 02-4084, 2002

CHAPTER
3

Preparing Yourself Mentally for the Task of Losing Weight

Information on how psychological factors influence a patient's weight should be an essential part of a weight-management program. Often, most of us shy away from matters related to our mental and emotional health. However, I believe there are two powerful influences that can interfere with your weight-loss and weight-maintenance efforts. They are stress from within, such as depression over your weight, and stress from the outside, such as pressure at work. Once again, along with the unseen metabolic pirate, these two strong influences are lurking in the background, eagerly waiting to snatch away your health. Don't let them win!

Accordingly, the purpose of this chapter is to bring to your attention several psychological roadblocks that could seriously interfere with your weight-loss and weight-maintenance efforts. Most likely, one or more of these roadblocks may be responsible for continued failure in your past weight-loss and weight-maintenance efforts. Such roadblocks can prevent you from adopting beneficial lifestyle behaviors that could improve your health. For these reasons, it is very important that you carefully read this entire chapter and answer all questions.

In this chapter you will learn practical pointers to reduce the stress from within caused by the three psychological roadblocks, and in the next chapter, practical pointers to reduce stress from outside pressures will be presented. The third step on your road to better health and fitness is to adopt a positive view of yourself and your weight to become psychologically healthy.

Identifying Three Psychological Roadblocks

The three psychological roadblocks to be identified in this chapter include low self-concept, body image, and low self-esteem. Such roadblocks can reduce self-confidence and retard self-improvement. See the "Evaluating My Psychological Health" on the following pages. Note that there is a section for each of these three concepts.

Write down the answers to the questions for self-concept, body image, and self-esteem and how you would rate each of the three concepts on a six-point scale and in the "Workbook of My Progress" in the appendix.

Because this evaluation is for your benefit, it is very important that you carefully read the questions so that the answers best reflect your feelings, not how you think others would expect you to answer. Based on your responses, you will be able to focus on those specific recommendations that best meet your personal challenges and preferences. *The six-point scales and questions for each of the concepts have been designed here to provide a relative evaluation from "lowest" to "highest" to determine your improvement regarding the concept, not as a medical diagnosis.*

Evaluating My Psychological Health

Section 1: Your Self-Concept

Rate your self-concept on a six-point scale, with one being lowest and six being highest, by considering the following questions. Write down "AG" if you agree with the question, "UN" if you are undecided, and "DG" if you disagree. For every *two* questions that you answer "agree," move one point up the scale:

1. I am a loving person because I can show affection through such actions as a smile, compliment, hug, or kiss.

2. I am sexually mature because I can both give and receive sexual pleasure.

3. I am a sociable person because I enjoy sharing news and activities with others.

4. I am appreciative of others because I value their presence in my life.

5. I am a caring person because, when needed, I give a helping hand or support to family, friends, and my community.

6. I strive to improve myself mentally because I continue to participate in such activities as reading, taking classes, or learning a craft or skill.

7. I am a good citizen because I participate in such activities as keeping abreast of local and world news and voting.

8. I am an honest person because I follow a moral code that discourages stealing and cheating.

9. I am physically active because I exercise thirty to sixty minutes at least five days weekly.

10. I am satisfied with my weight because I like what I see in the mirror.

Section 2: Your Body Image

Rate your body image on a six-point scale, with one being lowest and six being highest, by considering the following questions. Write down "AG" if you agree with the question, "UN" if you are undecided, and "DG" if you disagree. For every *one* question that you answer "disagree," move one point up the scale:

1. For the most part, I am dissatisfied with my physical appearance.

2. My physical appearance highly influences my self-concept (how I view myself as a person).

3. According to the popular one-through-ten physical attractiveness scale, I would rate myself low (less than five) because of my physical appearance.

4. My weight highly contributes to how I feel about my physical appearance.

5. I frequently feel hurt when I am teased, humiliated, or rejected because of my weight.

Section 3: Your Self-Esteem

Rate your self-esteem on a six-point scale, with one being lowest and six being highest, by considering the following questions. Write down "AG" if you agree with the question, "UN" if you are undecided, and "DG" if you disagree. For every *one* question that you answer "agree," move one point up the scale:

1. I accept myself, recognizing both my strengths and limitations.

2. I have faith in myself to obtain those things I value in life.

3. I have confidence that I can meet life's challenges.

4. I have self-discipline because I can refrain from those things that are harmful and pursue those things that are beneficial.

5. I am reliable because I do those things that I promise to do for myself and others.

Practical Pointers to Improve Your Self-Concept

Planning Activities

I recommend that you plan a variety of activities that can improve your self-concept. A practical step is to keep a calendar of events where you can plan and carry out specific activities. You may wish to purchase a calendar where the days have sufficient space to write the activity and its time and place. Or you may keep an ongoing log (date, activity, time, and place) by a method of choice and name it "Healthy Planning (Not If but When)." For the first two months of your weight-loss program, select one or two attributes (or characteristics), like *loving* and *sociable*, that you wish to improve. For months three and four, as well as five and six, continue with the same two attributes; continue with one attribute and select a new one, or select two new attributes.

The goal is to have these activities become part of your everyday routine. For those you marked as disagreed, plan an activity or two once or more weekly. For those marked as undecided, plan an activity or two every two weeks. It is highly recommended that you spend fifteen to twenty minutes on a weekend day to plan and think through the activities for the following week or two.

Other practical pointers include the following:

• Strive to fill your calendar with a balance of activities—those that are done for self-improvement and enjoyment and those that are done out of love and service to others.

• You may wish to have a balance in your activities by planning some activities that you do alone, but it would also be helpful to include activities that can be done with friends and family members, who can be supportive. They can often jump-start your enthusiasm when you are hesitant, as well as brainstorm new ideas for activities.

- It is best that you start with activities that are simple and then graduate to more demanding ones.

- Plan some activities that are familiar, some that are new, and some that are imaginative.

- Most of your activities should be action oriented (energy burning) and should remove you from the home.

- Have your activities include a variety of resources: bookstores and craft shops, libraries, the internet, professional workshops, and the like.

Recommended Activities

Activities to boost your self-concept for the personal attributes in (section 1) include the following:

1. Loving, Appreciative, and Sociable

   - Start with a smile, compliment, touch, hug, or kiss.

   - Next, offer to do a household, yard task, or errand otherwise done by another family member. If needed, offer to babysit or help a sibling with homework.

   - Take time with a loved one by visiting or by sharing activities, such as playing games or looking at family photos.

   - Plan to attend special outings with friends or family members, including activities like a day at the mall, sports events, or a visit to a museum.

2. Caring

- You may wish to start the activities listed under being loving, appreciative, and sociable.

- Start doing house and yard tasks or errands for elderly or handicapped neighbors.

- Volunteer to coach a sports team of interest.

- Volunteer at a local animal shelter.

- Volunteer, participate, or contribute to fundraising events or services of a charity or local organization of interest.

3. Sexually Mature

- In addition to sharing sexual pleasure, explore other romantic ideas. Periodically present your loved one with a special gift such as flowers, a card, or a poem.

- Plan a romantic candlelit dinner, a picnic for two in the park, or a quiet evening with music.

- A night at the movies, a play, or a concert is always well appreciated.

4. Mentally

- Try walking to a park or library and reading one or two chapters in a book of interest, reading one or two articles in a favorite magazine, or doing one or two crossword puzzles.

- Visit a local bookstore or library and scout out new fiction or nonfiction selections.

- Try auditing or taking a class (literature, creative writing, mythology, photography, etc.). Learn a new craft (knitting, crocheting, cross-stitch, pottery making, etc.) or a new hobby (gardening, woodworking, etc.). Search magazines and internet websites for new craft ideas, such as those presenting Home-Decorating Ideas.

- Explore a new skill (computer, self-defense, basic carpentry, cooking, sewing, quilting, etc.). If you love acting, join a local theater group.

5. Good Citizen

- Start with regularly keeping abreast of local and world news.

- Investigate candidates and issues related to voting, and always honor the law.

- Purchase or read at your local library magazines that provide news-and health-related articles. Reread the Declaration of Independence, the Gettysburg Address, and the Bill of Rights.

- Write your local or federal congressperson regarding issues of concern. Go online or visit museums or sites of historical importance.

6. Honest

- Since honesty has its basis in a moral code, you may wish to focus on spiritual growth, whether it is in God or a higher power.

- Start by attending a place of worship of your choice on a regular basis.

- Find a quiet place to read inspirational passages from a religious book of your choice.

- Visit a library or bookstore to check out new books on spiritual topics. Ask your librarian about authors who write inspirational novels.

- Join a Bible study group or choir.

- Volunteer as an usher, an assistant or teacher for Sunday school, or a leader for youth activities.

7. Physically Fit

- In chapter 9, based on your physician's approval, you will be setting goals and planning a physical fitness program.

- For the purpose of your calendar, you may wish to note activities such as your visits to a local health facility, swimming at the Y, or taking aerobic classes.

- Also, note on your calendar family-oriented physical activities, such as hiking or biking together or a family night out for bowling.

8. Weight

- In chapter 8, you will be selecting a diet plan that is nutritionally balanced and that will enable you to attain realistic weight loss and a healthy weight.

- Within your diet plan, select a variety of foods and beverages that will provide the nutrients that can support a healthy look to your hair, skin, and teeth (for that beautiful smile).

- Additionally, you will be asked to survey your favorite stores for lower-fat products.

- Also, visit your local library, a bookstore, or the internet to discover new low-calorie recipes.

- Plan to prepare some of these low-calorie recipes of interest.

- It is highly recommended that you involve family members, especially your children, in the above three activities, because they provide excellent opportunities for learning.

- You can use your calendar of events to plan such activities.

Regardless of how you rated your self-concept, I recommend that you keep such a calendar of events. Important to a healthy spirit is having something to look forward to, whether it is for self-improvement, for enjoyment, or as a service to others. Such activities focus your attention on the present rather than on past regrets or future concerns, while keeping you busy with constructive and rewarding activities. Healthy planning requires time and effort, but its beneficial results are worthwhile and rewarding to both you and your family. Strive to make the planning of worthwhile and satisfying activities a lifelong practice.

Practical Pointers to Improve Your Body Image

A Healthy versus an Unhealthy Perspective

I recommend that you acquire a healthy perspective concerning your weight. Many overweight and obese individuals desire to reduce their weight to "look better." However, when the expected weight loss is not achieved or when the weight that has been lost is regained, they are disappointed and feel defeated. The degree of these feelings depends on how many attempts they have made to shed the unwanted pounds.

Why? Most likely, it is a result of a person's psychological perspective. The four parameters that can shape this perspective include a person's self-concept, body image, physical appearance, and weight.

Review your responses to the first four questions in section 2. If you disagreed with these four questions, you have a healthy perspective, which includes the following:

- A healthy perspective is where all four parameters are in balance (no one parameter dominates).

- This perspective is constructive, being expressed by positive thoughts, emotions, and actions.

In contrast, if you agreed with one or more of these four questions, you have an unhealthy perspective, which includes the following:

- An unhealthy perspective is where the four parameters are out of balance (one or more parameters dominates).

- This perspective is nonproductive, being expressed by negative thoughts, emotions, and actions.

- This is especially true when weight is the overpowering parameter.

This evaluation was designed to help you realize the following:

- In addition to your physical appearance, you have many other personal attributes within your self-concept (physical, mental, and emotional), for example, participating in a sport you love, getting good grades, and caring for others, that are appealing. Such attributes can make you attractive, admired, and respected by others.

- Similarly, you have other physical attributes that can make you attractive to others, such as sharing sexual pleasure and being physically fit.

- Besides weight, you have other physical features that can make you attractive—for example, healthy hair and skin that shine, eyes that light up with interest and laughter, and a ready smile. All of these are universally appealing.

- Being overly critical of your weight can keep you from appreciating those features you like.

- More importantly, when weight becomes an overriding concern, it can distract you from realizing all the other personal attributes that make you the unique and beautiful person you are.

Keep in mind, it is not wrong to lose weight for the purpose of improving your physical appearance. However, strive for a healthy perspective, where weight loss is a target, not an obsession.

Positive versus Negative Wardrobe Selections

Concentrate on finding a look that is your very own. In a university class on fabrics, I learned a number of helpful tips related to wardrobe that can be recommended for overweight and obese individuals. I would like to share them with you:

- Select darker colors, because they have a slenderizing effect, such as black, navy blue, charcoal gray, dark green, or deep maroon.

- Avoid bold colors, because they draw immediate attention.

- Substitute bold colors with subdued and pastel colors.

- Stick with the smaller checks and prints.

- Bolder and larger designs not only catch attention but also magnify size. Select the thinner, vertical stripes in lieu of the broader, horizontal ones.

- Thinner, vertical stripes have a slenderizing effect, but they also focus the eye upon length rather than width.

When I was a chubby teen, the fashion rage of the day was stretch pants with stirrups for the feet. I tried on a black pair. When looking in the mirror, I was taken by surprise to see the noticeable slimming effect of such dark pants.

Accepting versus Rejecting Negativity Related to Excess Weight

Negativity directed toward the overweight and obese can produce and reinforce a poor body image and by doing so, threaten your weight-loss and weight-maintenance success.

The power of this negative influence should not be underestimated. Equally strong efforts described in the following practical pointers are required to counter this force.

Do not become mentally trapped in despair due to careless criticism from others. Consider the following:

- Past and present criticism, whether it is in the form of teasing, humiliation, or rejection concerning your weight, is a strong force in producing and reinforcing a poor body image.

- Such demeaning experiences can trigger the negative thinking that can result in unhealthy emotions and actions. Do not dwell on these past insults and criticisms.

- Most often, such critical comments and negative actions come from a person who is thoughtless or unkind or from a person who is prejudiced, judging you on the basis of socially derived notions about people who are overweight and obese.

- Though it is difficult, learn to disregard their comments and actions.

- Who would want to be with such negative and narrow-minded individuals?

- If this is unavoidable, such as with a family member or coworker, learn to tune them out.

- Just remember that your appearance is only a momentary target for their abuse, for they readily return to their own problems and concerns.

- Work hard to seek out old and new family members and friends who will be supportive and who share similar interests.

If you experience any demeaning remarks by a health professional, such remarks are uncalled for and unprofessional. Do not forgo medical attention you may require because of these remarks. If you encounter such insincere behavior, confront the professional by saying, "I didn't come for such remarks." All patients deserve respect.

Do not become discouraged with society's negative view of people who are overweight and obese:

- It is very important not to succumb to the media's unhealthy message that super thinness is the ideal standard for physical attractiveness.

- Stop comparing yourself with others, especially media stars.

- Ask yourself, "Is the thin look a significant measure that I would use in determining another's worth?" For most of us, it is not.

- Weight should not be the standard for judging another person's worth. This includes your worth as well.

- Compared to weight, being friendly, caring, reliable, and hardworking are heavyweights in terms of a person's being loved, accepted, and respected and in terms of being viewed as competent in the eyes of others.

Ladies, you do not need a pretty face and super-thin figure and gentlemen, a handsome face and buffed-up physique to be accepted and respected. It is the person's personality, talents, and commitments, not weight, that determine his or her ability to form loving relationships and accomplish that which is desired. Try to concentrate on those personal attributes that really make a difference to you and your loved ones.

Self-Approving versus Self-Critical and Defeating Thoughts

Replace self-critical and destructive thoughts about your weight, such as "I am too fat" and "I will not get a job," with self-approving ones, such as "everyone is special, including me," "I am unique in my own right," "my talents will help me succeed," and "I am healthy and capable." Start training your thinking to be positive, open, and assertive, especially in terms of your weight.

In cases when such negative thoughts become overwhelming, seek out a quiet place to meditate (chapter 4).

Constructive versus Destructive Emotions and Actions

Negative, weight-related experiences and self-criticism or criticism by others about your weight can trigger self-critical and defeating thoughts. Self-critical and defeating thoughts are not only personally painful and engender self-doubt, but they can also give rise to strong negative emotions that can result in destructive actions that include others as well. Depression and resentment can lead to withdrawal from others; anger can cause one to lash out at others; and frustration can result in becoming argumentative with others.

Call upon your inner strength and turn your attention to more constructive pursuits. Read a chapter or two in a favorite novel or magazine; watch a favorite or new video; complete a crossword puzzle; or work on a craft of interest. Concentrate on being positive. In other words, don't dwell on negative thoughts. Controlling your emotions and keeping busy are required to overcome the powerful pull of this negative thinking to promote psychological well-being.

Emotional Overeating

Depression, anger, frustration, and other strong emotions can trigger emotional overeating. Consider the following:

- In many cases, such emotional distress sends you automatically to the refrigerator or cupboard.

- Quite often, foods and beverages that are high in calories, sugar, and fat and that are easily available are chosen. This can lead to high calorie intakes and excess weight.

- When you are experiencing such emotional distress, pause for a few moments and breathe deeply to guard against reacting immediately to this emotional-driven impulse to overeat.

- In chapter 7, you will be introduced to the "energy gauge" and asked to post this on your refrigerator and cupboard.

- The posting of this gauge is to help you to stop and ask yourself, "Am I really hungry?" Probably you are not.

- Basically, the purpose of this gauge is to help you reduce unconscious or impulsive overeating.

- In addition, it reduces your reliance on external cues, such as food advertisements, that prompt you to eat, while encouraging you to become attentive to your inner feelings of being hungry or being full.

- Over time, focus on reducing this emotional overeating by becoming more in tune with such internal signals, until such conscious eating becomes second nature. In the meantime, concentrate on replacing these emotional impulses to overeat with more constructive actions that require physical activity and remove you from the home.

This impulsive overeating is triggered not only by emotional distress but also by everyday life-related stresses. In chapter 4, additional mental and physical relaxation techniques will be described that can be applied to both of these causes of overeating.

Examples of Experiences Involving Negative Thinking, Emotions, and Actions

Thus far, the practical pointers given above may seem to you to be abstract in nature. The following three examples will bring these abstract concepts down to earth. The mental and physical techniques described in the following chapter can also be used to reduce weight-related emotional stress.

Example A: A waitress at a local restaurant

Reason: I saw myself in my new bathing suit in the mirror.

Consider the following situation:

- Reactions: I thought, *I look like a beached whale. People will stare.* I became angry and frustrated and wanted to eat.

- Results: In the kitchen, I saw the energy gauge on my fridge. It reminded me to ask myself, "Am I really hungry?" I decided I wasn't. I remembered to do something constructive. I called my best friend to go biking, which made me feel calmer and in control.

- Reward: I rewarded myself by doing a cross-stitching project.

Example B: A clerk at a local grocery store

Consider this thought process:

- Reason: My aunt made a critical comment: "Boy, you're really getting pudgy."

- Reactions: I thought, *Those bulges are gross! Boys will think I'm unattractive.* I became depressed and resentful.

- Results: I took a few moments to meditate. This time helped me open my mind to focus on the positive personal attributes that are uniquely mine. My emotional turmoil subsided. I also remembered the importance of joining with supportive others. So I participated in a nature walk with friends, which reduced my stress and gave me peace of mind.

- Reward: We decided to play a game of miniature golf on Saturday.

Example C: A male accountant at a local business

Consider this scenario:

- Reason: At a party, one of my in-laws said, "Boy, have you packed on the pounds!"

- Reaction: I believed that everyone was focusing on my oozing flab. I became upset, embarrassed, frustrated, resentful, and angry.

- Results: I wanted to go to the snack bar and dig in and drown myself in beer. But I remembered to pause for a few moments to get a grip on my hateful feelings for him and myself as well. I also realized that he was right and I needed to learn how to eat more carefully and to increase my physical activity. As a result, I didn't do the uncontrolled bingeing that I had planned.

- Reward: I asked a couple of my guy friends to go golfing on the weekend, an activity I do like and have not done for some time.

Whenever you are confronted by negative weight-related experiences or comments, remember to take constructive action to control the emotional distress that is both physically and emotionally harmful.

When you become depressed, review all the above practical steps to improve your body image.

Practical Pointers to Improve Your Self-Esteem

On Your Pathway to Personal Growth

To improve your body image, you adopted a healthy perspective concerning your weight. By doing so, you can come to realize that acquiring personal happiness does not require a perfect weight. To improve your self-concept, you made a commitment to plan and carry out a variety of constructive activities, ranging from simple to more difficult. By doing so, you confronted new challenges, discovered special talents, learned new skills, and took pride in your accomplishments. Such activities can increase your self-motivation, discipline, and confidence. Standing by your commitments to do such activities can also demonstrate your reliability and patience, capturing the admiration and respect of family members, friends, coworkers, and your community. They bolstered your self-respect as well. All of these positive changes placed you on the pathway to personal growth, which is essential for self-acceptance and assurance. Self-acceptance and assurance are required for a healthy self-esteem and psychological health. Investing in your psychological health and a positive outlook for the future is a benefit not only to you but to your family as well.

Another practical way you can increase your self-esteem is to read and take to heart positive commitments for the day.

Write down these positive statements on a sheet of paper in large print. Place this list on your refrigerator to read before eating breakfast.

An example that you may use for the positive statements is included here. Use as a motto, "Filter out the negative, while focusing on the positive." Repeat these statements to yourself:

1. I have faith in myself and my abilities to acquire what I desire.

2. I have confidence in myself, because I can face and solve problems that arise in my life and make future plans, which I will accomplish.

3. I will be open to change.

4. I will join with others who have positive interests and goals.

5. I will be responsible for my actions, and if I don't succeed, I will rebound and try again.

Also, before going to bed, take a few quiet moments to think about the positive things you have done this day or the positive things that have happened to you or both.

Gather Your Supportive Troops

Be sure to include your supportive partner or support team. At your meeting(s), you can share and seek advice concerning your negative experiences. You can brainstorm ideas for constructive actions and rewards. You may wish to plan activities that you can do together. You will most likely have more fun and experience more progress in such a supportive setting. A balance of efforts that is based on both personal motivation and social support can be highly rewarding and productive. I would also recommend that you and your supportive partner or others review the practical pointers regarding body image discussed earlier in the chapter and especially focus on a healthy perspective.

Helping Your Child Become Psychologically Fit

Media and social messages promote the idea that being super-thin is required to be attractive, popular, and successful. As a result, an unhealthy focus on weight and dissatisfaction with their bodies occurs, especially among girls. This can trigger unhealthy eating practices.

It is important to be watchful of the dietary practices of children and teens, as well as the types of information they are exposed to through printed or internet information.

Work hard to convince your children, especially teens, that the media's message promoting super-thinness is an unhealthy ideal. Periodically remind your child or teen not to compare him or herself with others, especially with media stars. Rather, explain there is a healthy weight range for each individual. Emphasize that weight should not be the standard for judging a person's worth or acceptance. How can these healthy beliefs be reinforced by parental actions? To downplay weight as the central focus in the minds of children and teens, do the following actions often. Hug and kiss your children, and tell them that you love them, especially those who have a weight problem.

Compliment your child and teen on his or her beautiful smile, sharing with other children, being friendly, getting good grades, athletic ability, and so on. Strongly discourage weight-related criticisms and actions, especially among siblings. Assign each child or teen a small task, such as for the household or yard, and gradually add more difficult ones to promote confidence and a positive self-esteem. To show your respect for individuals of different sizes and shapes, point out important qualities in relatives and friends, such as caring, willingness to help, or being reliable.

Periodically reward your children and teens with a smile or praise for positive comments about others, regardless of the person's weight.

Concerning the psychologically based eating disorders, if you practice dietary restraint, yo-yo dieting (repeated cycles of gain and loss), or any other eating disorder, work hard to improve your own eating and activity practices, or seek professional help, along with your teen. Do not become an example or impose such unhealthy eating practices on your child or teen, whether or not he or she has a weight problem.

Become alert to whether your child or teen is overly concerned about or dissatisfied with his or her weight, becomes depressed or withdrawn, reduces food intake, or skips meals. In addition, carefully watch your children, especially teens, for signs of starving, binge eating, or vomiting after meals. These disorders are very serious and should be caught early. If you observe such practices, emphasize to your teen that good eating and activity practices can help prevent compromised health during the significant growth taking place in his or her life. If you see any evidence of such unhealthy behaviors being continued, contact your child's physician. Ask the physician to refer you to a professional experienced in the area of eating disorders.

Carefully read the following chapter on setting healthy goals for the family; it summarizes the eating and activity recommendations in specific detail, as presented in the previous chapters. Efforts to change unhealthy eating and activity practices will take time, effort, and patience, but they will be worthwhile, as they will ensure a happier and healthier family.

CHAPTER
4

Stress Management

Stress produced by pressures that are ever present due to today's fast-paced living can negatively affect your health, both physically and mentally, as well as your family and your work or school activities. These physical and mental symptoms can range from mild to severe. Stress can result in physical symptoms, such as headaches, ulcers, diarrhea, and heart problems, and mental symptoms such as depression, frustration, and anger.

In addition, stress can cause serious overeating and weight gain. It is recommended that you do not initiate a weight-loss program during extremely stressful episodes, such as the death of a loved one, divorce, or the loss of a job. If you have already started a weight-loss program, it is best that you delay such efforts until a less stressful time. The fourth step on your road to better health and fitness is to reduce the level of stress in your life to prevent illness.

Identifying the Causes of Stress

Before identifying the causes of stress, rate your stress level on the following five-point scale: 1, slightly stressed; 2, somewhat stressed; 3, fairly stressed; 4, moderately stressed; and 5, very stressed. *This scale has been designed here to provide a relative evaluation from "slightly stressed" to "very stressed" to determine your improvement in reducing stress, not as a medical diagnosis.*

Stress can be produced by personal, social, financial, and situational pressures. In many cases, stress results from being overbooked and overwhelmed by too many personal and social commitments.

- Personal responsibilities are commitments related to family, work and/or school, or church. Time for personal needs is required as well, including physical needs and establishing or maintaining relationships.

- Social obligations involve those that are made to relatives, friends, coworkers, and the community.

- Financial pressure could be due to not enough money, unemployment, or bankruptcy.

- Stressful situations could result from being trapped in heavy traffic, faced with long grocery lines, confronted by unexpected personal injuries or illness or those of a family member, or unplanned automobile or appliance breakdowns.

Simplifying Your Life

The media often refers to the present society as the prescription generation. Many individuals attempt to reduce stress by using prescription drugs or over-the-counter products. As with the supportive medications in chapter 2, such drugs and products can provide a temporary solution, but they do not target the cause of the problem. I believe that the most serious source of stress is that we crowd our schedules with too many activities and become overwhelmed when we do so. This ongoing pressure to respond to too many demands creates a frenzied way of life, characterized by an undercurrent of constant tension. We need to scale down our schedules to get rid of this buzz in our daily lives.

How? There is time that is devoted to family obligations (or for those we care about), such as birthdays, anniversaries, and holidays; for household and yard chores; for work and school (classroom and homework); and for church attendance, if desired. In addition to these stable commitments, there are extra activities that are related to these three areas, plus our interest in community events and organizations.

I recommend that you make a list of your extra activities in these four areas. Then participate in only one or two of these activities weekly.

This applies to individuals, parents, teens, and children. Examples include

- attending or participating in a sports event;

- going shopping at a mall or theatre to see a movie;

- attending or helping prepare a barbecue sponsored by your work;

- attending or being a volunteer at a fundraising event sponsored by a community organization; and

- attending or preparing a dish for a potluck sponsored by your place of worship.

Additional recommendations related to extra activities are as follows:

- Family household and yard chores should be shared by all members.

- If you do not believe in God or a higher power, select one or two organizations whose members are positive and whose purpose you support.

- Select extra activities that are meaningful to you and best match your interests and abilities, not based on pressure or approval or expected by others.

- You may wish to stagger some of the extra activities on a six-month or yearly basis—for example, volunteering at an animal shelter, joining a bowling league, or teaching Sunday school.

Of importance here is that by downsizing your schedule, your time can be focused on planning, shopping for, and preparing healthy meals and snacks and participating in a variety of physical activities, both on an individual basis and family centered.

If you are burdened with financial problems, seek help from an agency with experts experienced in such areas. Search out governmental and community programs for financial and energy assistance, medical and dental services, food pantries, or thrift shops.

Physical Relaxation Techniques

There are three types of physical relaxation techniques to be discussed here. These relaxation techniques can be done at home and at work.

Deep breathing is often recommended to reduce stress. In addition to using this technique at home and at work, try to apply it during a traffic jam or while waiting in a long line. Inhale deeply, and then exhale slowly. Continue to do so until you feel a quieting effect.

Another way to reduce stress is to become physically active. When you are feeling pressured, briskly walk for fifteen minutes during a break at work or when at home. Additional moderate-intensity activities are described in chapter 9.

Following are helpful exercises to reduce tension. For each exercise, stretch for a few seconds by counting up to three. When you return to an original position, relax for a few seconds. Be sure you feel a sensation of stretching. Do each exercise three to five times. Here are six specific muscle-stretching exercises to reduce tension, especially in the neck and shoulder regions:

- Gradually turn your head to the left until your chin touches your shoulder. Face forward. Repeat the same turning motion to the right.

- Move your head forward until your chin rests on your chest. Face forward. Repeat the movement backward.

- Lower your head to the left until your ear touches your shoulder. Face forward. Repeat the same lowering motion to the right.

- Stand with your arms at your sides. Gradually raise them until your palms come together over your head. Return to the original position.

- Raise both shoulders together until they reach your ears. Return to the original position.

- Raise your arms to shoulder level. Rotate both arms clockwise, return to the original position, and then rotate them counterclockwise.

Mental Relaxation Techniques

There are several mental relaxation techniques you may wish to try. Practice meditation in a quiet place without interruptions for fifteen minutes in times of stress. Make small visits to your dictionary, and make a list of positive words, such as peaceful, restful, contentment, or confident, that can be used alone or within a phrase, such as peaceful and calm or tranquil and content. While meditating, read from this list several positive words and phrases, and think of them in terms of the persons, things, or situations in your life.

Alternatively while meditating, you can recall a positive experience or a positive scene from a book, movie, or television program—for example, seeing a cloudless blue sky, hearing the splashing of gentle waves, feeling the soothing caress of a gentle breeze and the warm sunshine on your face and warm sand at your feet, while picnicking at a beach. Lighting a candle or listening to soft, instrumental music can enhance the effects of mediation.

Before going to bed, take a few minutes to do a brief meditation session, practice deep breathing, or do a few stretching exercises to help you acquire a restful sleep, which is important physically and mentally.

Alternatively, read a few scriptures from the Bible or your religious resource of choice or check with your librarian for authors who write inspirational novels.

Take advantage of all opportunities that can make you laugh, including watching television and movie comedies; reading newspaper comic strips or comic books; or selecting novels whose purpose is humor. It is very important that you select from the above physical and mental relaxation techniques those that best match your personal needs and apply them when confronted by stressful experiences.

An Example of a Patient's Experience

This patient is forty-six years old, a registered pharmacist, and married and has three children. He rated his level of stress on the five-point stress scale as a four at the beginning of his weight-loss efforts and two at six months. He listed three major stress-producing factors in his life and the mental and physical relaxation techniques he used to confront them, as follows:

1. For his very demanding job, he began to walk briskly for fifteen minutes on his break or do stretching exercises to reduce neck and shoulder tension.

2. Because he had too many personal and social demands, he downsized his schedule to only one or two extra activities in these areas.

3. To help him cope with heavy traffic on the way to work, he did deep-breathing exercises.

At this time, see your "Workbook of My Progress" for a strategy that you can plan to reduce stress in the appendix.

Gather Your Supportive Troops

When meeting with your supportive partner or support team, share ideas about removing extra activities, major causes of stress, and the mental and physical relaxation techniques to use.

Applying What You Have Learned

You have learned a number of practical steps to improve your self-concept, body image, and self-esteem (chapter 3) to reduce the stress caused by your emotional and physical reactions to self-criticism or the criticism by others concerning your weight. In this chapter, you have learned the organizational, physical, and mental techniques to reduce stress triggered by outside situations. I would recommend that you practice what you have learned from these two chapters for two or three weeks before beginning your weight-loss efforts. If you do so, these practical steps and techniques will be familiar to you so you can call upon them, if needed, during your weight-loss efforts.

CHAPTER
5 Basic Nutritional Facts

The information in this chapter is to promote five healthy goals—that is, the five Hs: a healthy weight, mind, dietary intake, eating practices, and physical activity. It is recommended that these healthy practices become lifetime commitments.

The information in this chapter focuses on important sources of key nutrients; explanation of nutrition labeling to compare foods and beverages in terms of calorie and nutrient content; and the role of dietary supplements.

The fifth step is to learn basic nutritional information to help you attain a healthy weight, mind, dietary intake, eating practices, and physical activities.

The Importance of Balance in Nutrition

Why is balance important? As previously emphasized, balance is the key to good health. Our bodies have many unique physiological and metabolic mechanisms, which respond to the stresses of everyday living to keep us healthy. They strive to maintain a state of homeostasis, or balance, in the body. In extreme situations, these mechanisms become overwhelmed, and we begin to experience health complications.

Extremes involving intakes and activity level can disrupt this homeostasis, resulting in unhealthy metabolic imbalances and consequences. Consider the following:

- Limited caloric intake can result in an underweight status, while an excess can produce obesity. Both a severe underweight status and obesity can interfere with the normal female hormonal balance, reducing the likelihood of becoming pregnant.

- Limited exercise each day can result in physical weakness and weight gain, while an excess can often cause hormonal abnormalities and weight loss.

- Limited amounts of vitamins and minerals can result in deficiencies, while excess amounts can cause toxicities. Excesses of vitamins and minerals can also result in harmful nutrient interactions and serious side effects.

The Energy-Producing Nutrients

What substances in food and beverages provide us with calories? The three nutrients in our diets that provide energy are carbohydrates, protein, and fats. Fat produces more than twice the number of calories than carbohydrates and protein per gram. This is the reason for the recommendation that when dieting, we need to watch how many fatty and fried foods we eat. A brief description of the sources of these dietary components is given here.

Carbohydrates include starches and sugars. Starches are present in breads, cereals, rolls, buns, crackers, and tortillas. They are also found in potatoes, dried beans and peas, rice, and pastas. Natural sugars occur in fructose in fruits and lactose in milk and milk products. Sugar is added to bakery products such as pastries, desserts, candies, jams, and jellies.

Complex carbohydrates, including fiber, are present in whole-grain breads and cereals, as well as fruits and vegetables.

Protein is found in meats, milk and milk products, eggs, dried beans and peas, and nuts and seeds.

Fats are found in margarines, butter, oils, salad dressings, nuts, and seeds. Fats are also present in meats, fish, dairy products, snack products, pastries, and desserts.

Types of Fats and Cholesterol and Sodium

The Properties of Fats

Polyunsaturated and monounsaturated fats occur naturally in foods. Although a small amount of trans-fats are present in food, the greater amount is artificially produced when vegetable oils are hydrogenated (adding hydrogen) to convert them to more solid fats.

Sources of Fats

Polyunsaturated fats include corn, soybeans, and other vegetable oils. The two essential fatty acids are present in such oils. Monounsaturated fats are present in olives, peanuts and peanut butter, and avocados and are included in peanut and olive oils. Omega-3 fats (a special group of polyunsaturated fats) occur in fish and fish oils, such as tuna and salmon.

Saturated fats are found in meats, dairy products, butter, lard, and palm and coconut oils. Trans-fats are present in hydrogenated margarines and shortenings. They are also present in bakery products, snack items, fried foods, and other products prepared with such fats.

Cholesterol and Sodium

Cholesterol is only present in animal products, being especially high in egg yolks and organ meats. It also occurs in meat and dairy fat. Sodium is found in table salt and salty foods. For the most part, snack, processed, canned, frozen, restaurant, and fast foods have a high sodium content.

Recommendations for Selecting Fats

Based on the above facts, some healthy selections can be suggested:

- As often as possible, select the foods and fats that have monounsaturated and omega-3 fats.

- Soft margarines are preferred over the more solid stick margarines, which have a higher percentage of trans fats.

Vitamins and Minerals

Vitamin A in the form of beta carotene occurs in dark green leafy vegetables and deep yellow (or orange) fruits and vegetables. Such vegetables include broccoli, spinach, greens, carrots, and sweet potatoes. Fruits include cantaloupe, peaches, and apricots. Beta carotene is converted to vitamin A in the body.

Vitamin C is found in citrus fruits and juices (such as orange and grapefruit), in melons (such as cantaloupe), and in berries (such as strawberries). Vegetables with vitamin C include green peppers, broccoli, brussels sprouts, cauliflower, tomatoes, and cabbage.

Folic acid (or folate) is present in dark-green leafy vegetables, such as broccoli and spinach, and orange juice. It is also found in fortified cereals and grains.

Iron is present in whole-grain, enriched bread, and cereal products. Iron occurs in dried fruits, such as raisins and prunes, and such vegetables as spinach and greens. When such foods are eaten along with a rich vitamin C source, absorption of iron is increased. Meat is a good source of iron because this iron is readily absorbed.

The best sources of calcium in the diet are milk and milk products. Calcium also has been added to some juices, candies, and calcium-fortified cereals. Check labels.

Are there advantages to acquiring vitamins and minerals from foods rather than from vitamin-mineral supplements? Definitely! Vitamins and minerals from supplements are not as effective in preventing disease or restoring health as those acquired from food. The important advantages are presented here.

- Health-Promoting Constituents: When you take such supplements in lieu of nourishing foods, such as fruits and vegetables and whole-grain products, you are excluding biologically active substances that are highly protective against cancer, heart disease, and stroke.

- Synergistic Effect: Food is a complex physical mixture of nutrients and other food components. These nutrients and food components often interact and produce a greater beneficial effect (a synergistic effect) above that when nutrients and food components are taken separately.

- Naturally Balanced Constituents: Also, this complex physical mixture of food can prevent harmful excess amounts that can occur when vitamins and minerals are taken alone.

Why Is Nutrition Labeling Important?

You can use basic nutrition facts to better understand nutrition labeling. Nutrition labeling established by the United States Department of Agriculture (USDA) enables you to compare the nutritional value of food and beverage products. You can then select those products that best meet your nutritional needs. When shopping, compare products with similar serving sizes. For example, it is easier to compare percentages of vitamins and minerals where both products have a serving size of a half cup rather than one being a half cup and the other one cup.

There are three sources of nutrition information on labels:

1. Commercial product labels list nutrition information, beginning with a list of the ingredients in descending amounts, with the highest amount listed first. For example, certain breakfast cereals, sodas and other sweetened beverages, flavored milks, and dessert-type products have a high content of sugar. Products that have sugar as one of the first three or four ingredients should be considered as having a high sugar content.

2. Look for special labeling. Families need to watch the amount of fat in their diets. Look for labels with lowered amounts of fat, starting with fat-free, then low-fat, and then reduced-fat. If a product is "light," it has a reduced number of calories.

3. Read the nutrition facts panel. Be careful because some packages or containers have more than one serving. I recommend that

you compare products with similar serving sizes. They should be lower in calories, be lower in total fat, have a higher percent of recommended levels of vitamins and minerals, have a higher fiber content, have a lower cholesterol content, and have a lower sodium content

Remember to stop to read and compare labels.

Dietary Supplements

As you peruse the shelfs of supplements, you will notice that they include several different types: vitamin-mineral and amino acid supplements, other dietary supplements, and herbal supplements.

Unlike drugs, remember that supplements can be marketed without proof of their safety, quality (contents), and effectiveness without prior approval of the Food and Drug Administration (FDA). For example, undesirable contaminants can be present in supplements, such as heavy metals like lead. If you have any concerns about a supplement's safety, such as possible contamination or adverse health effects, or wish to report a problem with the supplement, contact the FDA at 800-332-1088 or www.fda.gov/medwatch.

Supplements are appealing because they are thought to have magical powers. However, regarding effectiveness, in 2007, the Federal Trade Commission (FTC) that oversees marketing and advertising brought to our attention that a number of manufacturers providing weight-loss supplements were false, because they were ineffective in producing the weight loss claimed on the product label. Thus, dietary supplements can be risky not only in terms of safety and quality but also in terms of personal disappointment and financial loss due to a product's ineffectiveness.

If you decide to use a supplement, to reduce such uncertainties (safety and quality) surrounding such a product, I would suggest the organizations that independently test the supplement's safety and quality to evaluate the accuracy of the product's manufacturer. These organizations have seals of approval, which include the initials of the organization. Check your choice to see if it has a seal of approval.

In addition, when investigating a supplement, examine how much and what type of manufacturers' research supports the effectiveness of the product. Explore other internet resources for research regarding a given supplement.

Vitamin and Mineral Supplements

Healthy individuals who consume nourishing meals and snacks do not require a vitamin and/or mineral supplement. Remember the following when considering whether to take supplements:

- If you take a supplement, intakes from dietary sources, and fortified foods, the supplement should not exceed 100 percent of a vitamin's or mineral's recommended level. Check supplement labels.

- For adults, children, and teens who are on nutritionally balanced diets, consuming more than the recommended intakes of vitamins and minerals does not provide additional health benefits.

- The idea that one tablet is good, so two or more may be better is not valid.

- Excess can result in toxicity or unhealthy interactions between the supplement and other vitamins or minerals and prescribed medications.

- Often, a physician may recommend a vitamin and/or mineral supplement if there is a medical problem, like anemia, or an eating problem, like anorexia.

- In such cases, the amount of the vitamin or mineral may be higher than the recommended level when under medical supervision.

If you are taking a vitamin and/or mineral supplement that is effective and of good quality, continue with this product until it is no longer required. Additionally, strive to take this supplement in a consistent way, preferably with meals.

Precautions Regarding Dietary Supplements

There are several safety-related concerns regarding supplements that are summarized as follows:

- Not for All: As with drugs, there are individual differences in terms of which supplements are appropriate for an individual. Check with your physician.

- Negative Interactions: Supplements can interfere with the therapeutic actions of over-the-counter and prescription medications. For example, omega-3 (N-3) fatty acids in fish oil supplements should not be taken along with anticoagulant (anticlotting) medications. Why? Both of these reduce the body's ability to form blood clots.

- Inappropriate Use: Adult supplements of any type are not recommended for children and teens.

The best approach is before purchasing a supplement, you may wish to contact the FDA at the number given previously. It must be stressed here that before taking any supplement, contact your physician, who has your medical history. He or she can help you evaluate the product safety and quality in light of your individual medical history, including the drugs you are taking. Your physician can also monitor for any adverse effects that may have been unreported and determine whether the product is effective in terms of providing a sufficient amount of health benefits to warrant its expense. Registered pharmacists, registered dietitians, or public health nutritionists (if available) are valuable resources for information. Last, be sure to determine what the standard dosage or recommended level of the supplement is from such professionals.

Gather Your Supportive Troops

At your meeting(s) with your supportive partner or support team, you may wish to review the key nutrients and their sources. You may wish to exchange your experiences with the use of nutrition labeling and different dietary supplements.

Before Beginning Your Weight-Loss Efforts

I highly recommend that you survey your favorite grocery stores using nutrition labeling to guide your selection of healthy foods and beverages that you can use in your weight-loss and weight-maintenance dietary plans. For more detail, see your "Workbook of My Progress" described in the appendix.

CHAPTER
6   Determining What Is Right or Wrong with Your Dietary Intake

Concerning the calorie content of diets, individuals need to be instructed on how to modify their caloric intake to achieve a modest weight loss (chapter 8). The focus of this chapter is evaluating your intake of dairy products, fruits and vegetables, and whole-grain products, the food groups that are often neglected by many American adults. Your intake of alcoholic beverages will be considered as well.

The sixth step on your road to better health and fitness is to improve the nutritional quality of your diet.

Importance of Standard Measurement Sizes

Learning standard measurement sizes can enable you to better recognize appropriate portion sizes for your family. In the beginning, you may wish to measure the serving sizes of your foods and beverages. Alternatively, you could separate a standard nest of measuring cups and set of measuring spoons and display them in a place near the table where you can easily visualize them. This will aid you in learning how to eventually identify correct portion sizes.

The following points may be helpful:

1. Purchase a standard eight-ounce measuring cup or a standard set of measuring cups. Notice the markings on the standard measuring cups—one-fourth, one-half, three-fourths, and one cup.

2. Glassware comes in different sizes. To measure how much fluid your favorite glass or mug holds, fill a standard eight-ounce

measuring cup. For example, your mug may hold one and one-quarter cups or ten ounces of fluid. (Don't fill glassware to the top; you need to allow for spillage.)

3. You may use regular flatware teaspoons and tablespoons, but avoid using the larger serving spoons. If you wish to be more accurate, you can purchase a standard set of measuring spoons. For the purpose of the diet plans in this book, keep in mind that one cup is eight ounces, three-fourths of a cup is six ounces, and a half of a cup is four ounces.

Protective Constituents in Foods: Oxidants vs. Antioxidants

During the normal metabolism of nutrients from food, the body does produce "oxidants" (oxidative radicals). When larger amounts of food are consumed, more oxidative radicals will be produced. These oxidative radicals can cause destructive changes in cellular membranes (such as those of arteries) and cellular DNA. Such cellular damages are the underlining causes of several life-threatening diseases, including cardiovascular disease and cancer. Whole-grain products and fruits and vegetables contain certain vitamins and minerals (as vitamins E and selenium) and other plant constituents that can serve as "antioxidants" that prevent the oxidative damage to membranes and DNA.

Benefits of Whole-Grain Products

Whole grains (wheat, corn, oats, rye, and barley) contain endosperm, germ, and bran (including fiber). To produce refined flour, the germ and bran portions are removed, leaving the "starchy" endosperm. Such processing removes not only fiber but also many disease-preventing constituents.

Complex carbohydrates (present in whole grains and fruits and vegetables) are slowly digested and absorbed, resulting in a gradual rise in blood glucose and insulin levels. In contrast, foods with a high content of sugar, including all sweets, are rapidly digested and absorbed. This results in a rapid rise and early peaking of blood glucose and insulin, an unhealthy metabolic state. This unhealthy state could eventually cause an increased risk for type 2 diabetes.

Both whole-grain products and fruits and vegetables contain complex carbohydrates in the form of soluble and insoluble fiber. Because this fiber provides bulk and a lasting feeling of being full within a meal and between meals, it is more likely that reasonable amounts will be consumed. In contrast, because foods high in sugar content are highly flavorful and readily available, an excess of calories can be consumed before you feel full. Because of this, whole-grain products and fruits and vegetables can assist you with your task of weight management.

The above differences underscore the need to replace foods high in sugar content with whole-grain products. Such positive properties (along with antioxidants, vitamins and minerals, and other plant constituents) can reduce your risk for disease.

Several servings of whole-grain products are recommended daily. For example, for breakfast, try a whole-grain cereal or a whole-grain toast. For lunch, fix a sandwich with whole-grain bread or a whole-grain bun or have cheese and peanut butter with a whole-grain bagel. For supper, include whole-grain pasta or wild rice. Remember a whole-grain bagel or bun can be considered as two servings.

Try adding cinnamon to your whole-grain cereal or toast and to other foods as well. Adding one-fourth to one-half teaspoon of cinnamon daily to foods can help maintain a healthy blood glucose level. Additionally, you may wish to try cereals that already contain cinnamon.

Benefits of Fruits and Vegetables

I strongly recommend that you consume a variety of fruits and vegetables daily.

There are a number of protective constituents in fruits and vegetables that can lower your risk for disease. There are a number of vitamins and other plant constituents that act as antioxidants:

- beta carotene (or vitamin A): Present in dark green leafy vegetables and deep yellow (orangish) fruits and vegetables, described shortly

- lycopen: Present in deep red fruits and vegetables as in tomatoes and tomato products (paste and sauce)

- vitamin C: Present in citrus fruits and juices and other fruits and vegetables, described shortly

- folic acid (folate): Present in dark green leafy vegetables, like kale and spinach, and fortified cereals

- vitamin E: Present in whole-grain products and vegetable oils, such as corn

Several plant constituents are protective because they rid the body of foreign substances, such as carcinogens (cancer-producing):

- sulfur-containing constituents: Present in the onion family and garlic

- sulfur-containing constituents: Present in cruciferous (or cross-like vegetables), such as broccoli, cauliflower, brussels sprouts, cabbage (coleslaw, cooked cabbage, or sauerkraut), and bok choy

It is important to realize that there is a high content of protective constituents under the skins of fruits and vegetables. Because of this, eat your fruits and vegetables, such as apples and potatoes, with the skins intact. Recall that vitamins and minerals provided by food are more effective in preventing disease than in their supplement form. From our discussion concerning the protective value of whole-grain products and fruits and vegetables, it is safe to say that nature with its unique wisdom has provided us with the best medicines to prevent disease, such as heart and lung disease, high blood pressure, and stroke. It is now up to us to take advantage of it.

Evaluating Your Dietary Intake in Terms of Nutritional Quality

To do this, refer to "Evaluating the Nutritional Quality of My Diet" on the following pages. As you read through this evaluation, write in your workbook your answers to question 3 for the sources of calcium, fruits and vegetables in general, fruits and vegetables high in vitamins A and C, whole-grain products, and alcohol intake in terms of the number of days you met the recommendation. Behind the number of days, answer yes if you met the recommendation for all seven days or no if you did not.

Evaluating the Nutritional Quality of My Diet

Sources of Calcium

1. Three sources high in calcium are recommended daily.

2. Serving sizes include the following:

   - 8 ounces of milk, including those modified for dieters with lactose intolerance

   - 6–8 ounces of yogurt

   - 2 ounces of cheese

   - fortified foods, such as cereals and juice, that have 30 percent or more of the daily recommended level of calcium

   - supplements that contain at least 300 milligrams of calcium daily

   - It is recommended here that you meet this dietary recommendation by means of dietary sources or by a combination of dietary and supplement sources rather than by supplements alone.

3. In a typical week, how many days do you meet this recommendation, from zero to seven?

Fruits and Vegetables

1. Five or more servings of fruits or vegetables are recommended daily.

2. Serving sizes include the following:

   - 4 ounces of juice

   - a small piece of fruit

   - 1/2 cup of fruit

   - 1/2 cup of cooked vegetables

   - cup of raw vegetables

3. In a typical week, how many days do you meet this recommendation, from zero to seven?

Fruits and Vegetables High in Vitamin C

1. One serving of a fruit or vegetable high in vitamin C is recommended daily.

2. The serving sizes are the same as those for fruits and vegetables above. Sources include the following:

   - citrus fruits and juices, such as orange and grapefruit

   - berries, such as strawberries, and other fruits, such as pineapple

   - broccoli, brussels sprouts, cabbage, cauliflower, green pepper, greens, and tomatoes

3. In a typical week, how many days do you meet this recommendation, from zero to seven?

Fruits and Vegetables High in Vitamin A

1. One serving of a fruit or vegetable high in vitamin A is recommended daily (or a minimum of three times weekly).

2. The serving sizes are the same as those for fruits and vegetables above. Sources include the following:

   - apricots, peaches, and cantaloupe

   - broccoli, greens, spinach, carrots, winter squash, and pumpkin

3. In a typical week, how many days do you meet this recommendation, from zero to seven?

Whole-Grain Products

1. Three or more servings of whole-grain products is recommended daily.

2. Serving sizes include the following:

   - slice of whole-grain bread or 1/2 a whole-grain bagel or bun (hamburger or hot dog)

   - 3/4 cup of ready-to-eat whole-grain cereal or 1/2 cup of cooked whole-grain cereal

   - 1/2 cup of whole-grain pasta or wild rice

   - crackers or snack products (check product label for serving size)

3. In a typical week, how many days do you meet this recommendation, from zero to seven?

Alcoholic Beverages

- It is recommended here that men and women have no more than one alcoholic beverage daily. In table 5, information about alcoholic beverages is given.

Table 5: Alcoholic Beverages

Alcoholic Beverages Considered as One Drink
12 ounces of beer
1–2 ounces of distilled spirits
5 ounces of wine (or a 10-ounce wine cooler)

- Based upon your food records, how many days of the week did you meet this recommendation from zero to seven?

Gather Your Supportive Troops

At your meeting(s), you and your supportive partner or support team may wish to share the results of the evaluation of your dietary intake. Also, if available, exchange recipes that include or that could be revised to include the fruits and vegetables high in vitamins A and C and whole-grain pastas or rice.

CHAPTER
7
Determining What Is Right or Wrong with Your Eating Practices

Why has there been a dramatic increase in the number of overweight and obese US adults in recent years? Recall that many American adults are consuming too many calories and expending too few, which can result in an undesirable weight gain over time. There are a number of modern-day eating practices contributing to this unwanted gain. These eating practices will be discussed here.

The seventh step on your road to better health and fitness is to improve your eating practices.

Eating Practices of Concern

Do you try to control or reduce your weight by bingeing (a bout of eating a large amount of food), seriously restricting your intake, vomiting, diuretics, laxatives, or excessive exercise? If you are doing one or more of these practices, you most likely have a serious eating disorder. Ask your physician to refer you to a professional experienced in the area of eating disorders.

Over time such practices, particularly vomiting or using diuretics or laxatives, can result in serious medical complications. For example, stomach acid from consistent vomiting could injure the esophagus and can corrode your teeth.

Recommended Frequencies for Eating Practices

For the eating practices in this chapter, recommended frequencies are presented. These recommended frequencies apply to both individuals and families.

The recommended frequencies for the first three eating practices are expressed in terms of at least 90 percent of the time (on a weekly basis). For example, let us say that you are eating three meals and one snack daily for a week. This is twenty-eight meals and snacks (m/s) and 90 percent would be twenty-five of these twenty-eight m/s. Ask yourself, "Did I meet the recommended frequency?" If you did not, think about the percentage you are doing presently. Use the following percentages as a guide: 89 to 80 = 24 to 22 m/s; 79 to 70 = 21 to 20 m/s; 69 to 60 = 19 to 17 m/s; 59 to 50 = 16 to 14 m/s; 49 to 40 = 13 to 11 m/s; 39 to 30 = 10 to 8 m/s; 29 to 20 = 7 to 6 m/s; 19 to 10 = 5 to 3 m/s; and 9 to 0 = 2 to 0 m/s. For example, 60 percent would be seventeen meals and snacks weekly and 45 percent would be twelve meals and snacks weekly.

The remaining eating practices are expressed in terms of "a recommended number of days" on a weekly basis. If you do not meet the exact recommended number of days, think about the number of days, zero to seven, that you are presently meeting the recommendations.

Undoubtedly, these frequencies and recommended number of days will require significant changes for you. Because of this, gradually change an unhealthy eating practice until you meet its recommended frequency or number of days.

Write down in your workbook the eating practices that met the 90 percent recommendation and the estimated frequency for those practices not meeting this recommendation. Likewise, for the remaining eating practices, write down the number of days that the recommendation was met for the specific eating practice.

Eating Regular Meals and Snacks

Unhealthy Eating Practice

When eating on the run, you are more likely to select fast food or convenience items containing a high amount of calories (highly sweet or high in fat).

Recommendations

It would be better to pace your day to prepare regular nourishing meals and snacks. However, if you are rushed, make a conscious effort to select the healthier fast food or convenience items. On a weekly basis, strive to have regular meals and snacks at least 90 percent of the time.

Becoming Tuned In to Your Internal Feelings of Hunger and Being Full

Unhealthy Eating Practice

Impulsive and erratic eating should be avoided, because such practices can lead to overeating of less-nourishing meals and snacks.

Recommendations

Ideally, the best approach is to rely on internal feelings of hunger and being full to control food intake:

- Responding to only internal feelings is an effective way of controlling intake, by reducing the risk of impulsive or erratic eating.

- Also, strive to resist responding to such external cues as TV or advertisements about food or the desire or pressure to start or stop eating just because others do.

It is recommended here that a regular pattern of balanced meals and snacks with a variety of foods and beverages be reinforced by becoming in tune with your appetite-related internal feelings. However, relying solely on internal feelings is difficult for some dieters. Because of this, at the beginning of your weight-loss efforts, it is best to rely on and adhere to the recommended portion sizes of your weight-loss plan. As you begin to lose weight, work hard to become sensitive to your internal feelings of hunger and being full.

How internal feelings of hunger and being full can fit into a meal and snack pattern is explained in the following paragraphs.

Just how is appetite regulated? Consider the following:

- The empty fuel gauge in a car indicates to the owner that there is a need for gas to power the engine.

- Similarly, an empty stomach indicates to your brain the need for food and the calories it provides to power your body.

This guide provides a practical tool to help you become more aware of your internal feelings of being hungry and being full. This practical tool, your energy gauge, is a practical tool that uses the stomach as your energy gauge.

In this case, there are several degrees of being empty or the need for calories:

- First, the levels of hunger (indicating the need for calories) are represented by readings ranging from -1, meaning slightly hungry, to -3, very hungry.

- Second, the state of being no longer hungry, but not yet full, is represented by the reading of 00.

- Third, the levels of fullness (recognizing the receipt of calories) are represented by readings ranging from +1, meaning slightly full, to +3, meaning very full.

On a weekly basis, work hard to become more sensitive to your internal feelings of being hungry or full for meals and snacks at least 90 percent of the time.

Your Energy Gauge

- +3: Very full and should be avoided. If this occurs, take a leisurely walk.

- +2: Full, means stop eating.

- +1: Slightly full, means you should continue to eat.

- 00: No longer hungry, but not yet full, means you should continue to eat.

- -1: Slightly hungry, means you should continue to eat or start to eat lightly.

- -2: Hungry, means you should continue to eat or start to eat moderately.

- -3: Very hungry and should be avoided. If this occurs, eat slowly, at a steady pace, and moderately.

- Lightly could mean either by reducing the number of food and beverages normally eaten at a given meal or snack or by eating only half portions of the food and beverages normally consumed.

- Moderately could mean consuming the food and beverages normally eaten at a given meal or snack in appropriate portion (or serving) sizes.

- Take a second serving only if you feel hungry.

Reducing Your Portion Sizes

Unhealthy Eating Practice

Many restaurants, fast-food establishments, and so on offer larger portion sizes, such as super-packed sandwiches, larger packages of fries or ounces of beverages, and the like. Because of widespread and persuasive advertising, such products are accepted and purchased without question.

Recommendations

It is very important to pass on such products and select the regular or smaller-size meals/drinks. At home, eat the recommended serving sizes for foods and beverages (chapter 8). If you remain hungry, take a second serving, starting with a tablespoon. Keep these things in mind:

- Pay close attention to the recommended portion (serving) sizes on commercial product labels.

- Replace larger dinner plates, soup and cereal bowls, glasses (tumblers), and cups (mugs) with smaller ones.

- For snacks, use a small plate or bowl, custard cup, eight-ounce margarine tub, or a small baggie for chips or popcorn (preferably low fat or whole-grain).

On a weekly basis, strive to eat appropriate portion sizes for each meal and snack at least 90 percent of the time.

Increasing Family Meals

Unhealthy Eating Practice

When you eat meals and snacks outside of the home, they are quite frequently less healthy and in large portion sizes. Popular selections purchased away from home have higher calories, sugar, fat, cholesterol, and sodium.

Recommendations

You have the opportunity to prepare more nourishing meals and snacks. Strive to vary the settings for your family meals. For example, transport family meals to a local park, beach, lakeside, or your backyard. Share family meals with one or more neighbors by having a backyard potluck or barbecue. Keep the following in mind:

- A recommended goal is to have five or more family meals weekly. Family meals provide not only the opportunity to prepare healthy foods but also the time to communicate with each other.

- Strive to prepare healthy lunches for work three or more days weekly.

Reducing Your Pace of Eating

Unhealthy Eating Practice

A fast pace of eating can result in eating too much and gaining unwanted pounds.

Recommendations

Recommendations to help you slow your pace of eating include the following:

1. Take smaller bites, and chew each bite thoroughly.

2. Set down your fork or spoon between bites periodically.

3. Pause a few minutes within the meal.

Set your pace of eating so that major meals each day last between twenty and thirty minutes.

Reducing Your Intake of High-Calorie Foods

Unhealthy Eating Practice

Nutrient-rich products are low in fat and high in protein—that is, low-fat dairy items; lean meats, fish, and poultry; whole grains; and fruits and vegetables. High-calorie or nutrient-poor products are high in fat and salt (chips, pretzels, etc.) or high in fat and sugar (pastries, desserts, and other sweets). Keep the following in mind.

- Because nutrient-rich foods have a higher protein, fiber, and water content and because they are digested and absorbed more slowly, these foods have the ability to delay hunger.

- Because high-calorie products are highly flavorful and readily available, individuals quite often consume excessive amounts of such products, adding extra weight over time.

- This can place them on the pathway to obesity.

Recommendations

High-calorie products do add variety and pleasure to everyday meal and snack patterns:

- Keep in mind that all types of food and beverages in appropriate amounts can fit into a nutritionally balanced diet.

- Appropriate portion sizes and moderation (how often eaten) are key in keeping the calories from high-calorie foods within reasonable limits.

Remember—do not consistently (to a great extent) replace nutrient-rich products with high-calorie ones.

In addition, check product labels for calories per serving and recommended serving sizes. You may wish to make a list of the serving sizes of your favorite products just in case you desire to make them from scratch following a recipe. To further assist you with reducing your intake of high-calorie foods, practical suggestions include the following:

1. Slowly reduce the purchase of high-calorie products.

2. Then store those purchased items out of reach.

3. To reduce the temptation to overeat, confine such products to small containers (such as small baggies, custard cups, and eight-ounce margarine tubs, etc.).

The best suggestion is to allow a high-calorie food in an appropriate amount at one meal or snack no more than three days weekly.

Reducing Your Intake of High-Calorie Beverages

Unhealthy Eating Practice

High-calorie sweetened beverages include regular soft drinks, fruit drinks, Kool-Aid, and so forth. Coffee and tea that are highly sweetened with sugar or honey (more than one teaspoon) can be considered a high-calorie beverage. High fructose corn syrup (HFCS) (containing both fructose and glucose) is the preferred sweetener for most soft drinks. Check the list of ingredients on product labels for sweetened beverages and other commercial products for the presence of HFCS.

Popular soft drinks have an average of 160 calories per can. Remember the following:

- Table sugar (sucrose) contains fructose, which is bonded to glucose.

- However, during digestion the bonds are broken, giving rise to a mixture of fructose and glucose, like that found in HFCS.

- Thus, one serving of a HFCS soft drink would contain an equivalent of eight teaspoons of sugar.

- In addition, both fructose and glucose cause dental decay.

Recommendations

Both adults and children will benefit from reducing their intake of soft drinks and other sweetened beverages. It is strongly recommended that you do the following:

- Do not consistently (to a great extent) replace nutrient-rich beverages with high-calorie ones.

- Try to replace soft drinks and other sweetened beverages with water or juice.

- For those who are drinking high-calorie beverages, such as soft drinks, be careful not to increase your food intake, especially high-calorie foods. One Sunday, my family and I went to a buffet-type restaurant for lunch. I noticed a customer selecting a diet soft drink. However, for dessert, she selected a piece of chocolate cream pie. Unfortunately, the diet soft drink does not cancel the large amount of calories from the chocolate cream pie.

- It is recommended here that dieters who prefer sweetened beverages should consume no more than one cup (eight ounces) or one can (twelve ounces) of such beverages or two cups of coffee and tea that are highly sweetened with sugar or honey (more than one teaspoon) daily.

Reducing Eating in Rooms other than the Kitchen and Dining Room While Doing Other Activities

Unhealthy Eating Practice

This practice is notorious for being a situation that promotes overeating.

Recommendations

The ideal way to control such overeating is to eat all meals and snacks in the kitchen or dining area without participating in any other activity:

- However, realistically, adults and children enjoy eating a meal or snack in a recreation or family room, while watching TV, working on the computer, or reading.

- If you give way to temptation, doing such practices occasionally would be all right, but keep them to a minimum because they could lead to overeating.

- Instead of grabbing a bag of chips or package of cookies, select lighter and more nutritious meals and snacks. Use smaller containers, such as a small cereal bowl, custard cups, eight-ounce margarine tubs, or small baggies.

- Such practices not only help cut calories but also prevent you from overeating while your attention is focused elsewhere.

- It is recommended here that you work hard to keep this unhealthy eating practice to no more than three days weekly.

Decreasing Meals and Snacks Taken in Fast-Food Establishments and Restaurants

Unhealthy Eating Practice

Many popular selections at such eateries are high in calories, total fat, saturated fat, cholesterol, and sodium.

Recommendations

To prevent eating such excessive amounts of calories and fats, the following "select the smart way" tips are recommended when eating out at restaurants (buffet, by menu, or cafeteria-style) and fast-food establishments:

- Look for lighter or portion-controlled meals, such as heart-healthy, lighter-fare, mini meals, and so on.

- Instead of receiving it before the meal, request that a bread, roll, or chip basket be served along with the meal.

- For salads, ask for the lower-fat type variety of salad dressings to be placed on the side in a separate container.

- Avoid or select only a few items from the appetizer platter, because they are usually deep fat fried or have a high fat content.

- Select vegetable or broth-type soups over creamed ones.

- Choose baked, roasted, or grilled meats and fish over fried ones.

- Avoid selections served with heavy gravies, specialty sauces, cheese, or creamed sauces.

- Opt for a baked potato rather than mashed ones with gravy, french fries, hash browns, potato chips, and the like.

- Select green beans, carrots, or other green vegetables over corn, peas, lima beans, baked beans, or other starchy vegetables.

- Choose toast or bread (preferably whole-grain), an english muffin, a light roll, or a bagel instead of a specialty bread (like banana bread), muffin, biscuit, crepe, croissant, or any type of pastry.

- Request a low-fat variety milk, diet soft drink, water, juice, coffee, or tea over a regular soft drink, shake, high-caloric coffee-type beverage, alcoholic beverage, or any type of sweetened beverage.

- Pass on desserts because most of them are high in fat and sugar. Wait until you get home, and have some low-fat frozen yogurt, low-fat ice cream, fruit, and so forth.

- For sandwiches, opt for roasted or grilled chicken, turkey, fish, or lean beef in lieu of fried ones, bacon, or luncheon meats that tend to be high in fat (such as bologna or salami).

- Top off your sandwiches with mustard, ketchup, pickles, lettuce, tomatoes, bean sprouts, or other vegetables rather than mayonnaise, specialty sauces, tartar sauces, butter or margarine, and the like unless they are a lower-fat variety.

- For tacos, order those with lettuce and tomato, while avoiding those with sour cream and guacamole.

- Try to avoid larger or supersize portions. At an unfamiliar place, if larger portions are served, remember to share part with another or pack some away in a container to be eaten at a later time.

- At buffet-type restaurants, remember to take appropriate serving portions and second helpings only if you really feel hungry. If temptation over comes you, take a smaller portion of a salad, vegetable, or fruit.

It is strongly advised that you do not eat more than two days weekly at restaurants and fast-food establishments. This applies to takeout food and deliveries as well.

Reducing Emotional Overeating

Unhealthy Eating Practice

Emotional overeating can be triggered by strong emotions (anger, frustration, depression, etc.).

Recommendations

By becoming aware of these problematic times, you can be on guard against them. Remember the following:

- In situations when you are so stressed or emotionally upset, you may overeat without thinking.

- To prevent overeating at these times, your energy gauge, posted on your refrigerator or cabinet door, can serve as a signal to remind you not to automatically open the door.

- Pause for several minutes to study the different levels of hunger and being full on this gauge, and focus on your internal feelings.

- Ask yourself, "Am I really hungry, or do I want to eat because I am emotionally upset?"

- If you do feel hungry, decide at what level and eat according to the dietary recommendations given on the gauge.

- If you discover that you are not hungry, don't hesitate. Take constructive action.

- The best strategies to prevent overeating include becoming engaged in some type of physical activity or becoming involved in some constructive activity that may better appeal to you at the time (craft, novel, etc.).

These activities can replace or dispel the destructive physical and mental reactions caused by strong emotions. It will take practice and patience over time for you to distinguish your physical feelings of hunger and being full from the psychological need to eat caused by strong emotions or by environmental forces, such as social pressure, advertisements, and so on. Remember the following:

- Post lists of physical activities and/or other constructive activities by your energy gauge.

- All of the above recommendations can be applied when you are bored or become stressed.

- Over time, strongly strive to avoid such emotional overeating at any time.

Specific Circumstances

Reducing Your Overeating on Holidays and on Vacations

Do you have a problem with overeating on holidays or on vacations?

On these occasions, dieters who monitor or keep track of their food and beverage intakes are more likely to control their calorie intake. To do this, you may wish to use the log approach (chapter 6) or the practical form that tracks dietary intake (chapter 8). This recommendation also applies when you are home all day.

During vacations, such monitoring may be difficult. Alternatively, you may wish to monitor your food and beverage intake mentally as you progress through each day.

Most hotels and lodges have refrigerators in their rooms. Purchase and store healthy foods and beverages in such refrigerators. For breakfast, opt for cereal and a low-fat variety of milk. For meals and snacks when you are vacationing, take foods like peanut butter and crackers, small boxes of cereal, fruit, and so on. Include bottled water or a thermos filled with your favorite beverages. Backpacks are perfect for carrying such items.

Try hard to eat the majority of your meals and snacks in this fashion. By planning and controlling your intake, you can eat more healthily for less money. The money you save by making your own meals and snacks can be spent on additional entertainment, souvenirs, and the like. In addition, to work off calories consumed, plan vacations that are highly active, such as walking, hiking, swimming, and so on.

Reducing Your Overeating on Weekends

To better control your overeating on weekends, review your three-day log (chapter 6), and ask yourself these questions that compare intakes for weekend days versus weekdays:

- Are you eating more calories?

- Are you eating more meals and/or snacks?

- Are you eating more high-calorie foods?

- Are you eating more high-calorie sweetened beverages?

- Are you eating out more at restaurants and fast-food establishments?

By identifying the above problem areas, you can be on guard against them. By answering these questions, you can also better plan your meals and snacks to correct the overeating problem(s). Also, at noneating times, keep busy with other constructive activities, especially those that require actively moving or those that require your hands to be occupied.

Gather Your Supportive Troops

At meeting(s), you and your supportive partner or support team may wish to exchange thoughts about the different unhealthy eating practices and their recommendations. I strongly suggest that each of you make a list of the ten recommended frequencies and the recommendations given to correct them and the five questions regarding weekend versus weekday intakes. You may wish to use a blank sheet of paper and a black, felt-tip pen or a computer means of your choice to write these recommendations in large print. Post them on a cabinet or on the refrigerator as a quick daily reminder. These recommended frequencies are abbreviated as follows:

Ninety Percent of the Time (on a Weekly Basis)

1. Eat regular meals and snacks.

2. Respond to your appetite-related feelings.

3. Eat recommended portion sizes and slow down the pace of eating.

Number of Days Weekly

1. Prepare family meals five or more days per week.

2. Prepare healthy lunches for work three or more days per week.

3. Have only one high-calorie food no more than three days weekly.

4. Have only one high-calorie beverage daily.

5. Eat in other rooms doing an activity no more than three days weekly.

6. Avoid emotional overeating every day.

Weekend versus Weekday Intakes

1. Do you eat more calories?

2. Do you eat more meals and/or snacks?

3. Do you eat more high-calorie foods?

4. Do you drink more high-calorie, sweetened beverages?

5. Do you eat more outside of the home?

At this time, go to your workbook and write your results for the recommended frequencies and questions as described in the appendix

CHAPTER
8 Selecting a Weight-Loss Plan

When calories consumed are less than calories expended, you can reduce your weight. However, there are a number of biological factors, including genetic, metabolic, and hormonal factors, that can determine how much weight is lost. Instead of an ideal weight, these biological influences determine a range of weights that dieters can achieve. In some cases the dieter may be unable to reach the normal weight range. If this occurs, a more realistic goal is to strive to have your blood pressure and blood levels of glucose, LDL-c, HDL-c, and triglycerides within the normal range at the lowest weight you can obtain.

In addition, dieters often desire a higher percentage of weight loss than the recommended 10 percent. However, even though such weight losses can be achieved, they are rarely maintained. It is important to appreciate smaller weight-loss changes, such as the 10 percent, because such change can provide beneficial health effects and can be used as a criteria for success. The eighth step on your road to better health and fitness is to select a weight-loss plan that best matches your needs to reduce your weight wisely.

Advice about Pregnancy and Weight

Excess weight can cause physical difficulties for the mother and her infant during and after birth. If you have a weight problem, try to lose as many of the excess pounds as possible before getting pregnant. When pregnant, be sure to follow the weight gain and physical activity recommendations for each trimester recommended by your physician. Also, work hard to follow the dietary recommendations for pregnant women. Weight reduction should be delayed until after your baby is born. You may wish to read the information that identifies unhealthy eating practices and how to correct them (chapter 7), because they can add many extra calories to your intake, especially how to reduce your intake of high-calorie foods and beverages.

Smoking and Weight Control

Smokers are often reluctant to stop smoking, because they are afraid of gaining weight after quitting. It is important to realize that smoking is not a wise way to control weight. It is not prudent to initiate both weight-control and smoking-cessation programs at the same time. Whether you stop smoking before or after your weight-loss efforts, be watchful of high-calorie foods (all sweets and salty snacks) and high-calorie beverages (soft drinks and other sweetened beverages). As emphasized previously, these products are highly flavorful and readily available, encouraging an excess intake. Be careful not to swap one addiction for another.

Selecting a Weight-Loss Plan

For most overweight and obese individuals, I would recommend the following:

- The length of the weight-loss period is six months.

- Because your calorie intake is lower than your normal intake, ask your physician about a vitamin and mineral supplement.

- If you have insurance to do so, ask your physician to refer you to a registered dietitian or a public health nutritionist for advice and support on a regular basis.

- Have a six-month maintenance period before embarking upon further weight loss.

Because everyone's medical history and present medical profile are different, seek the approval of your physician for the weight loss and maintenance plans you will be following. The National Institutes of Health and the National Heart, Lung, and Blood Institute within the US Department of Health and Human Services, and North American Associates for the Study of Obesity recommend

"Diets containing 1,000 to 1,200 kcal/day should be selected for most women; a diet between 1,200 kcal/day and 1,600 kcal/day should be chosen for men and may be appropriate for women who weigh 165 pounds or more, or who exercise."[1] Intakes of less than 1,000 calories are not recommended because they are too restrictive and require close medical supervision.[1] Concerning these recommendations, you may wish to take the following steps.

To determine your present calorie intake, it is important that you keep a three-day log of your food and beverage intake and the subsequent five steps related to this log in your workbook. Select the two weekdays and one weekend day that best reflect your typical intake. This log will help you select a weight-loss diet that will best match your personal energy needs in terms of being workable and sustainable. In addition, by doing this three-day log, you can compare it with your selected weight-loss plan to identify problematic eating practices.

To receive the full benefit of this log, it is important that you complete your log of intake in an open way. Be careful of the pitfall of under-reporting. Try not to reduce your eating over the three-day period, and try not to avoid the high-caloric foods (such as snack foods and sweets) that you may normally consume. Remember the following:

1. For each day, include in your log the date; the specific meal or snack, such as lunch and a midafternoon snack; the specific food or beverage; the amount of the food or beverage; anything added to the food or beverage, such as margarine, salad dressing, or sugar; and how the food is prepared, such as baked or fried (amount of fat used). For example see "1,200-Calorie Weight-Loss Plan" on the following pages.

2. For food items that have more than one component, like a sandwich or casserole, estimate the amount of each component. For example, a ham sandwich with cheese would list two slices of whole wheat bread, two ounces of ham, one ounce of cheese, and two teaspoons of mustard. This applies to commercially produced meals as well. See also "Special Considerations" in the following pages.

3. Carefully read over "Serving Sizes for the Weight-Loss Plans" on the following pages.

4. Determine for all meals and snacks for each of the three days the number of servings you are presently consuming for the different food groups except for the meat and alternatives group, which should be noted as *number of ounces*: dairy products (milk and yogurt); meat and alternatives (eggs, cheese, peanut butter, and dried beans or peas); fruit group; vegetable group; grain group (breads, crackers, cereals, and pastas); fat group; and other group (snack products, desserts, and other sweets). For this latter group, write down the size of the dessert (such as a two-inch-square brownie), number of cookies, or number of chips. Check product labels for serving sizes. If homemade, check the label of a similar product. For sweetened beverages, use the serving sizes of a twelve-ounce can for a soft drink and an eight-ounce cup of other sweetened beverages. Serving sizes of various alcoholic beverages appear in chapter 6. When deciding on the number of serving sizes, an example is given here. The serving sizes for cooked cereals and pastas is half a cup. If you were to eat one cup, this would be two servings.

5. Then, for *each food group,* add the number of servings for the three days and divide by three (round off to the nearest whole number). For example, you have eaten eight servings from the bread group on day one, ten servings on day two, and seven servings on day three. This would be twenty-five divided by three, giving an average of about eight servings daily.

Compare the average number of servings from each of the food groups you are presently consuming with the number of servings given for the 1,000- to 1,600-calorie weight-loss plans (see "Weight-Loss Plans by Calorie Level" on the following pages). Select the weight-loss plan within the calorie range recommended for you that would be most reasonable and the one you would most likely be continued. For example, male dieters may favor a 1,500- or 1,600-calorie plan. Larger male dieters who are eating larger amounts of food may even consider a weight-loss plan between 1,700 and 2,000 calories.

It may be helpful for you to join with other family members who also wish to lose weight when keeping your three-day logs. For example, a husband and wife are working together to determine their present intakes by keeping their logs on the computer.

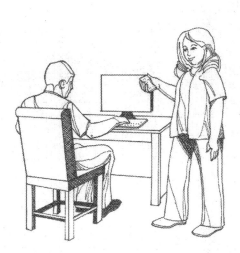

Precautions to Take during Your Weight-Loss Experience

Before embarking on your weight-loss program, the following important precautions need to be considered:

- During the course of your weight reduction, you may experience shifts in body water, which could result in a daily weight gain or loss of as much as two pounds. Do not be alarmed or discouraged with such a temporary gain. This does not represent an increase in fatty tissue. Keep your confidence intact, and continue your dietary and physical activity programs.

- At a point during the weight-loss period, dieters will experience a leveling in their weight loss—for example, a weight loss remains the same for three weeks. This phenomenon results because the body is equilibrating energy balance in response to changes in dietary intake and physical activity. At this point, you will need to adjust your caloric intake and diet plan to lose more weight. It is recommended that you reduce your intake and diet plan by increments of two hundred calories per day to jump-start the weight-reduction process again.

- If you stray from your weight-loss plan for a few days, do not criticize your weight or get discouraged. Do not say, "I have blown it, so I might as well stop my dieting efforts." Put a halt to this negative thinking, and restart your weight-loss efforts.

Weight-Loss Plans

Such plans range from 1,000 to 2,000 calories. See "Serving Sizes for the Weight-Loss Plans" and the "Weight-Loss Plans by Calorie Level" on the following pages. Serving (or portion) sizes play a significant role in controlling your calories.

Serving Sizes for the Weight-Loss Plans

Dairy Products

- One serving is eight ounces (one cup) of fat-free or 1 percent milk or six to eight ounces (three-quarters or one cup) of fat-free or low-fat yogurt.

- If 2 percent milk is preferred, count it as two servings of milk plus one serving of fat (two for one) in the dietary plan.

- The third serving can be two ounces of cheese, considered here as a meat alternative.

Meat and Meat Alternatives

- For meats, determine the amount after cooking and after removing bones, skin, and fat from the edges of meat. When cooked, four ounces of meat equals three ounces.

- An average portion of meat and an alternative is two or three ounces. This could include one of the following:

  o 2–3 ounces of poultry, meat, or fish

  o 2–3 ounces of sandwich meats

  o 2 ounces (1/4 cup) of tuna (water-packed or drained of oil)

  o 2–3 ounces of cheese

- An ounce of meat or an alternative can include one of the following:

  o 1 hot dog or 1 egg

  o 1 tablespoon of peanut butter

  o   1/2 cup of dried beans or peas

- Consider the size of a three-ounce patty, stack of thin slices, or a piece of meat as being four inches by three inches and a half inch thick. Examples include half a chicken breast; a regular-size hamburger, tenderloin, or pork chop; or a chicken or fish fillet.

- In addition, consider a chicken wing as one ounce and the leg and thigh as two ounces.

- Two ounces of cheese is two thin slices or the size of a two-inch-square chunk.

When meat and meat alternatives with a higher fat content are consumed, count this as one serving of the following plus one serving of fat in the dietary plan:

- each ounce of prime cuts

- each ounce of other meats high in fat (meatloaf, ground beef, bacon, etc.)

- each ounce of sandwich meats (bologna, pastrami) and one hot dog

- each ounce of the popular cheeses, such as cheddar

- each ounce of fried chicken or fish

- each egg scrambled or fried

- each tablespoon of peanut butter

- because of the high fat content, whether it's one, two, or three ounces or tablespoons, consume only one or two servings of such foods no more than twice weekly

Fruits and Vegetables

One serving of fruit is equal to the following:

- 4 ounces juice

- a small piece of fruit

- 1/2 cup berries or other fruits

- 1 cup melon

- 1/4 cup dried fruits

One serving of vegetables is equal to the following:

- 1/2 cup cooked vegetables

- 1 cup chopped raw vegetables or sticks

- 1 cup leafy raw vegetables (lettuce or spinach)

- 3/4 cup vegetable juice

Quite often, corn and potatoes are preferred, especially french fries, which have a higher fat content. Count each small serving or package of french fries as one serving of vegetable *plus* one serving of fat in the dietary plan. Such vegetables as corn, potatoes, peas, and lima beans contain a higher carbohydrate content. Because of this, it is best to offer these vegetables at mealtime only three or four days a week. Instead, you may wish to have a colorful vegetable plus a serving of a whole-grain pasta or wild rice.

Grains (Breads, Cereals, Pastas, and Other Grain Products)

One serving (preferably whole grain) is equal to the following:

- slice of bread or small roll

- 1/2 hamburger or hot dog bun

- 1/2 small bagel (one ounce) or 1/2 english muffin

- 1/2 cup cooked cereal, rice, or pasta

- 3/4 cup (1 ounce) of ready-to-eat cereal (lower added sugar preferred)

- 5–6 small or 3–4 large crackers

Fats and Oils

One serving is equal to the following:

- 1 teaspoon margarine, butter, mayonnaise, or vegetable oil

- 1 tablespoon salad dressing, cream cheese, or sour cream

Other Foods and Beverages

Some foods and beverages contain very few calories—that is, fewer than twenty-five calories per serving. Such foods and beverages can be included in the weight loss plan without considering them in the total daily intake of calories. These include condiments, such as mustard and ketchup; coffee, tea, or diet soft drinks; and certain fat-free products. Check product labels for calories per serving and serving size.

Weight-Loss Plans by Calorie Level

Note: The numbers given under the food groups represent number of servings, except for the meat and meat alternatives group, which represent ounces. Use the "Serving Sizes for the Weight-Loss Plans." The third serving of a calcium-rich source could be two ounces of cheese, which, for the purposes of these dietary plans, is included under the meat and meat alternatives group.

1,000 Calories

2 servings dairy

4 ounces meat or alternatives

3 servings of fruit

2 servings vegetables

4 servings grains

2 servings of fat

1,100 Calories

2 servings dairy

4 ounces meat or alternatives

3 servings fruit

2 servings vegetables

5 servings grains

2 servings of fat

1,200 Calories

2 servings dairy

5 ounces meat or alternatives

3 servings fruit

2 servings vegetables

6 servings grain

2 servings fat

1,300 Calories

2 servings dairy

6 ounces meat or alternatives

3 servings fruit

2 servings vegetables

6 servings grain

3 servings fat

1,400 Calories

2 servings dairy

6 ounces meat or alternatives

3 servings of fruit

2 servings vegetables

7 servings grains

3 servings of fat

1,500 Calories

2 servings dairy

6 ounces meat or alternatives

3 servings fruit

2 servings vegetables

8 servings grains

3 servings of fat

1,600 Calories

2 servings dairy

7 ounces meat or alternatives

4 servings fruit

2 servings vegetables

8 servings grain

3 servings fat

1,700 Calories

2 servings dairy

7 ounces meat or alternatives

4 servings fruit

3 servings vegetables

9 servings grain

3 servings fat

1,800 Calories
2 servings dairy
7 ounces meat or alternatives
4 servings fruit
3 servings vegetables
10 servings grain
4 servings fat

1,900 Calories
2 servings dairy
7 ounces meat or alternatives
4 servings fruit
3 servings vegetables
11 servings grain
4 servings fat

2,000 Calories
2 servings dairy
8 ounces meat or alternatives
4 servings fruit
3 servings vegetables
11 servings grain
5 servings fat

An Example of a 1,200-Calorie Weight-Loss Plan

For an example of a weight-loss plan, see the "1,200-Calorie Weight-Loss Plan" on the following pages. Remember the following:

- This plan has three meals and one snack.

- The snack may be a midmorning, midafternoon, or after-dinner snack.

- For the other weight-loss plans, you can add the necessary number of food groups to this dietary plan until they match the number of food groups given for the specific weight-loss plan.

- You can distribute the foods and beverages according to any type of meal and snack pattern that would best meet your individual preferences.

- The foods and beverages given on the plan are only examples.

- Exchange these for foods and beverages for those of preference.

1,200-Calorie Weight-Loss Plan

Here are the recommended servings per food group:

- 2 servings dairy

- 5 ounces meat or alternatives

- 3 servings fruit

- 2 servings vegetables

- 6 servings grain

- 2 servings fat

Breakfast Sample Menu

1 grain	3/4 cup unsweetened cereal, bagel (1 ounce), or 1 slice toast
1 milk	1 cup 1 percent milk or 6 ounces fat-free yogurt
1 fruit	1/2 cup orange juice, small banana, or medium peach
1 fat	1 teaspoon soft margarine for the toast

Lunch Sample Menu

2 grain	2 slices bread, 1 bun, or bagel (2 ounces)
2 meat	2 ounces lean sandwich meat, 2 ounces lower-fat cheese, or 2 tablespoons of reduced-calorie peanut butter
1 vegetable	1 cup carrot sticks, celery, or broccoli (raw)
1 fruit	1/2 cup apple juice, 1 small orange, or 1/2 cup pears
1 fat	1 teaspoon soft margarine for the vegetables
other foods	2 teaspoons of mustard

Dinner Sample Menu

1 grain	1 slice bread, 1 small roll, or bagel (1 ounce)
3 meat	3 ounces chicken, beef, pork, or fish
1 vegetable	1/2 cup green beans, spinach, etc.
1 vegetable	1 cup tomato wedges
1 fat	1 teaspoon soft margarine for the vegetable
1 milk	1 cup 1 percent milk or 6 ounces fat-free yogurt
other	1 or 2 tablespoons of fat-free salad dressing for tomatoes

Snack Sample Menu

1 grain	4 whole wheat crackers
1 fruit	1 small apple, 1 cup cantaloupe, or 1/2 cup strawberries

Selections and Preparation Tips

1. As often as possible, it is best to choose lean cuts of meat, lean hamburger, and low-fat luncheon meats, hot dogs, cheese, and peanut butter.

2. Prepare meats by baking, grilling, or broiling. Fry only occasionally.

3. Try to eat a variety of colorful vegetables (for example, red, deep yellow or orange, or green). These vegetables have a higher content of vitamin and minerals and protective substances that can keep you and your family healthy.

4. Fresh, frozen, and canned vegetables may be selected (although canned vegetables have a higher salt content). If canned vegetables are preferred, drain off the salty liquid and lightly rinse the vegetables with water.

5. Avoid fruits canned in heavy syrup.

6.   Among the six servings of grain products, strive to include three or more whole-grain products daily. Gradually introduce whole-grain products—eating too much at one time can cause digestive upsets. This also may apply to too many fruits and vegetables.

7.   Select fat-free or lower-fat margarines, salad dressings, mayonnaise, sour cream, and cream cheese. As often as possible, focus on the monounsaturated fats, such as olive and peanut oils.

8.   If you have a problem with too much sodium, lightly salt food while cooking or preparing or at the table, but not both. Always remember to taste the food first, and then lightly salt or use a nonsalt seasoning, if needed.

9.   Many snack foods, processed foods, frozen foods, and restaurants/ fast-foods are high in sodium content. Check product labels for the amount of sodium per serving. Consider products high in salt if the amount of sodium is 500 or more milligrams per serving.

Special Considerations

The following recommendations can be applied to foods and beverages that are prepared at home or at restaurants, fast-food establishments, or delis or that are commercially frozen or canned products.

How can dishes containing a number of ingredients (such as casseroles, chili, soups) be included in a dietary plan? If homemade, divide the measured amount of each ingredient by the number of servings the recipe suggests. Consider only those ingredients that contribute the most to the recipe. For such dishes, a recommended serving is one cup. For example, one cup of macaroni and cheese or a tuna casserole may contain about three-quarters of a cup of noodles and one ounce of tuna or cheese. Count this dish as having two servings from the grain group and one serving from the meat group.

Keep in mind that uncooked pasta doubles in size when cooked; for example, one cup uncooked becomes two cups cooked. For similar commercially prepared dishes, do your best to determine the amount of each ingredient. Check product labels for number of servings per container and serving size.

Likewise, for commercial meals and products (such as pizzas, tacos, hamburgers) determine the amount of each component. For example, a cheeseburger would contain one bun (two servings from the grain group), three ounces of hamburger, and one ounce of cheese (four servings from the meat group). Mustard, ketchup, and pickles are "free."

Count a meal of three ounces of turkey, half cup dressing, and half cup green beans as three servings of meat, one serving of grains, and one serving of vegetables.

Recommended Eating Practices to Improve While Reducing Your Weight

There are four recommended eating practices that involve calorie-costly foods and beverages. Such foods and beverages can add more variety and pleasure to your weight-loss plan. It is best to select those foods and beverages that have 250 calories or less (check nutrition label for calories). The information that can help you include the high-calorie foods and beverages into your plan are given below. For each food and beverage within a recommended eating practice that has the following characteristics, do the following:

- 100 calories or less, count as one serving of the grain group

- 101 to 150 calories, count as two servings of the grain group

- 151 to 200 calories, count as two servings of the grain group plus one serving of the fat group

- 201 to 250 calories, count as two servings of the grain group plus two servings of the fat group

1. Reduce your intake of high-calorie foods (all sweets and salty snack products) to one meal or snack no more than three days weekly. See nutrition label for serving sizes.

2. Reduce your intake of high-calorie beverages (a 12-ounce can or 8 ounces of a soft drink, 8 ounces of a sweetened beverage, or two cups of coffee or tea with more than one teaspoon of honey or sugar) (a teaspoon of honey or sugar has 20 calories) to a meal or snack no more than once daily.

3. Reduce your alcohol intake. I recommend one drink daily for both men and women. Select from:

    •   4 ounces of dry red or white wine or 1 ounce of a single liquor

    •   preferably, a 12-ounce can of light beer or 10 ounces of a light wine cooler

    •   12-ounce can of beer, 10-ounce wine cooler or 2 ounces of a mixed liquor drink

4. Reduce your intake at a restaurant or fast-food establishment to a meal or snack no more than two days weekly

    •   Work hard to choose the healthier selections as described in chapter 7.

    •   Search the internet for your favorite fast-food establishment. Write down your favorite high-calorie foods and beverages and their calories and healthier replacements and their calories.

    •   Write down the above information as described in your workbook in the appendix.

It is important to realize if you eat two or more of the high-calorie foods and beverages daily, you will be replacing too many of the nourishing grain products, especially if they are whole-grain items. I would advise you to have only one high-calorie item daily or two if their calories do not add up to more than 250 calories.

There are several other recommended eating practices to consider:

- Remember to stick to the recommended serving sizes given in your specific weight-loss plan.

- As you reduce your weight, concentrate on your internal feelings of hunger or being full.

- If needed, slow your pace of eating until major meals last between twenty to thirty minutes.

Recommended Physical Activity While Reducing Your Weight

For overweight and obese dieters, I would recommend starting with walking. Details about moderate-intensity walking are provided in chapter 9. Begin to exercise gradually. Keep the following in mind:

- At the beginning to three months: Walk for thirty minutes, five days weekly (could be in three ten-minute walks or two fifteen-minute bouts).

- Three to six months: Walk for forty-five minutes, six days weekly (could be in three fifteen-minute bouts).

- Six months and beyond: Walk for sixty minutes, seven days weekly (could be in three twenty-minute or two thirty-minute bouts).

Although these recommendations may be appropriate to many dieters, be sure to develop a physical activity plan that best matches your personal needs, including the advice of your physician and your preferences. Concerning the stretching and strengthening activities (chapter 9), I would recommend waiting until your maintenance period to begin these activities when you do not have to focus on applying the many recommendations given in chapters 1 to 7.

Planning Healthy Meals and Snacks

A recommendation here is to plan healthy meals and snacks. Set aside time (an hour or so on the weekend) to plan the meals and snacks for the following week and its grocery list. When planning your meals and snacks, keep variety, moderation, and balance in mind.

If you plan for meals and snacks acquired from fast-food establishments and restaurants (eaten at home or at the site), include the healthier selections based upon the nutrition fact sheets for fast foods (obtained at the site or from the internet) and healthy selections on the restaurants' menus. Remember that for restaurants and fast-food establishments, strive to keep the number of meals at such places to no more than two days weekly.

Keep Your Menu Planning Simple

- To assist you with this, refer to the example "General Menu Ideas and Related Grocery List" on the following pages.

- Record your menu plans in a spiral notebook or by a computer means of choice, using a similar format to the above example.

- This recording will enable you to reuse the same menu ideas at a future date, saving you time and effort. Such menu plans can also help trigger new menu ideas.

- Based on your specific diet plan, you can create your own menu ideas.

For most meals, strive for nutrition balance, including a protein food (meat or dairy or both); a fruit or vegetable or both; grain foods (such as cereal, bread, or roll, especially the whole-grain types); and a fat, such as margarine, salad dressing, or sour cream. It is strongly advised that you focus on making your meals and snacks attractive by including foods with different colors, textures, shapes, and tastes. For example, serve low-fat milk with a baked chicken breast, wild rice, mixed carrots and peas, and a small lettuce and tomato salad with low-fat ranch dressing. For dessert, provide a fruit cup or artificially sweetened Jell-O containing multiple types of fruit.

Are You Guilty of Shopping While Hungry and Eating While Cooking or Preparing Food?

When you shop when hungry, you are more likely to purchase unnecessary, high-calorie, and less-nutritious foods. The best approach is to take time and plan your meals and snacks. From this plan, create a shopping list, and strive not to deviate from it. By doing so, you are more likely to make wiser, healthier food choices.

If you eat while cooking or preparing food, try to resist such temptations. If you do need to check the flavor, learn how to just taste, not sample what you are preparing.

Allow sufficient time to prepare healthy meals and snacks. Use your menu plans as blueprints for preparing healthy foods and snacks. Keep in mind that such blueprints are not written in stone. Be flexible. For all of us, there will be unexpected circumstances that can interfere with your plans. Plan ahead by having healthy foods and beverages on hand that can be easily prepared when time is limited.

The best approach is to keep meals and snacks simple. Use heavy sauces and gravies only occasionally. For your meals, consider four items: (1) protein foods (meat and dairy); (2) vegetables, including starchy (like potatoes and colorful vegetables); (3) bread and other grains (especially whole-grain breads, rolls, etc.); and (4) a small amount of fats (margarine, sour cream, etc.). Also, fruit and fruit salads make simple and wonderful desserts and snacks. Additionally, when planning favorite dishes such as meatloaf and casseroles prepared in the oven or chili, soups, or stews prepared in the crock pot, double the recipes so you can freeze half of the dish to be served at a later time. When preparing some recipes, you may wish to exchange regular sugar with a sugar substitute.

It is best to prepare your favorite dishes, such as casseroles, from scratch, using ingredients that have lower fat, sugar, and sodium content. This can be true for other recipes as well.

Remember—as often as possible, make meals family meals. Make a strong effort to have all family members eat together at least five days weekly.

Creating Your Grocery List

Based on your menu plan, the next step is to develop a grocery list. Do not forget to include ingredients that will be required for old and new recipes that are used in your menu plans. Include your list behind each related menu plan in your notebook. Such grocery lists will reduce impulse shopping that generally results in the purchase of unhealthy foods and beverages.

Also, try hard each week to cut out coupons from local newspapers and keep store flyers, taking advantage of in-store bargains. Another resource is to search the internet by product name or company to check for available coupons.

General Menu Ideas and Related Grocery List

Mon	Tue	Wed	Thur	Fri	Sat	Sun
Breakfast	**Breakfast**	**Breakfast**	**Breakfast**	**Breakfast**	**Breakfast**	**Breakfast**
Cereal*	Bagel*	Cereal*	Toast*	Cereal*	Bagel *	Waffle*
Milk*	Yogurt*	Milk*	Jam	Milk*	Yogurt*	Syrup
Banana *	Peach*	Banana*	Margarine	Banana*	Peach*	Cantaloupe
Coffee	Coffee	Coffee	Coffee	Coffee	Coffee	Milk
Lunch	**Lunch**	**Lunch**	**Lunch**	**Lunch**	**Lunch**	**Lunch**
Turkey	Tuna	Ham	Cheese *	Tuna	Turkey	Ham
Bread**	Bread**	Bread**	Crackers*	Bread**	Bread**	Bread**
Lettuce *	Celery*	Carrots*	Lettuce*	Carrots*	Lettuce *	Carrots*
Tomato*	Carrots*	Margarine	Tomato*	Olives	Tomato*	Mustard
Ranch	Mayo	Pears*	Ranch	Mayo	Ranch	Pears*
Juice *	Juice*	Juice *	Juice *	Juice*	Juice *	Juice *
Dinner	**Dinner**	**Dinner**	**Dinner**	**Dinner**	**Dinner**	**Dinner**
Chili	Mac/ch *	Tacos	Pork chops	Catfish	Burger	Chicken
Saltines	Lettuce*	Chips	Potato*	Corn*	Bun**	Wild/rice*
Carrots*	Tomato*	Salsa	Roll*	G beans*	Catsup	Broccoli*
Margarine	French	Celery*	Spinach*	Margarine	Peas*	Margarine
Milk *	Milk *	Milk *	Milk *	Milk *	Milk *	Milk*
Snack	**Snack**	**Snack**	**Snack**	**Snack**	**Snack**	**Snack**
Apple*	Sherbet	Grapes*	Fruit/salad	Apple*	Grapes*	Popcorn

Also, jot down favorite recipe ingredients and planned selections from fast-food establishments and restaurants to be visited:

1. For macaroni and cheese, use 1 percent milk, American cheese (lower-fat), and macaroni.

2. For chili, use ground round, chili beans, onions, chili powder, and low-sodium tomato juice.

3. For fruit salad, use sugar-free cherry Jell-O with banana and light whipped topping.

4. For fast foods, eat tacos.

From your above menu ideas, use the following:

1. For milk products, use 1 percent milk and fat-free yogurt.

2. For meat and substitutes, use the following:

   A. boneless, skinless chicken breasts, ground round, pork chops, and catfish

   B. low-fat processed sandwich meats (turkey and ham) and cheese (low fat)

   C. water-packed tuna

   D. chili beans

3. Fruits:

   A. apples, bananas, cantaloupe, grapes, and peaches

   B. canned pears

   C. calcium-fortified orange juice

4. Grains:

   A. bread—whole wheat bread, pumpernickel or rye bagels, and whole wheat rolls

   B. cereals and grains—Shredded Wheat, Raisin Bran, wild rice, and macaroni

   C. crackers and snacks—whole wheat crackers, taco chips (baked), and low-fat microwave popcorn

   D. starchy vegetables—corn, peas, and potatoes

5. Vegetables:

   A. to cook—broccoli, green beans, spinach, and low-sodium tomato juice

   B. raw—carrots, celery, lettuce, tomatoes, and onions

6. Fats:

   A. olives

   B. lower-fat margarine spread (30 to 50 percent vegetable oil)

   C. low-fat mayonnaise (or Miracle Whip) and low-fat salad dressings (ranch and french)

7. Dessert—sherbet

8. Other foods:

   A. beverages—coffee and sugar-free soft drinks (occasionally)

   B. fats—low-fat cream cheese (for bagels), light whipped topping, and nonstick cooking spray

   C. light or sugar-free items—light jam, sugar-free syrup, sugar-free cherry Jell-O, sugar-free gum, and sweetener

   D. seasoning—chili powder

   E. other—bread-and-butter pickle slices, ketchup, and salsa

9. Frozen foods and entrees—8- to 11-ounce frozen meals or entrees (<350 calories).

The Importance of Monitoring Your Dietary Intake and Weight Loss

The extent and consistency of self-monitoring of dietary intake (or tracking) highly influence your amount of weight lost. A "Weekly Tracking Record of Food Groups" has been included on the following page so you can mark off the foods and beverages as they are being consumed throughout the day. This is a simple and a practical way to monitor the number of food groups. This record is particularly helpful for those individuals whose meal and snack patterns greatly differ from the sample pattern.

In addition, it is important to monitor your weight loss to determine the effectiveness of your weight-loss plan. I recommend that you keep a daily log of weights (the date and weight) in addition to recording it for a week. For this purpose, you can keep a weekly record of weight loss, see "Weekly Weight Checks." Keep in a notebook your weekly dietary tracking record and your log of daily weights and "Weekly Weight Checks."

Weekly Tracking Record of Food Groups

Instructions: Record the number of food groups given in your specific weight-loss plan. Then, use a tally or X mark for each food group that you consume during the day. In a notebook, keep copies of this tracking record. This also applies to a log of daily weights and a weekly weight check form to be described shortly. For vitamin C–rich fruits and vegetables, mark with a colored pencil or crayon in orange, vitamin A in green, and whole-grain items in brown. Place a green X by the days that you follow your weight-loss plan.

List	Number	M	T	W	Th	F	Sa	S
Milk or yogurt								
Meat/ other								
Fruit								
Vegetable								
Grain								
Fat								

Weekly Weight Checks

Instructions: Keep a daily log of your weights (date and weight). Include this ongoing log of weights and this weekly check form along with your dietary tracker record.

Week	Weight	Week	Weight
1		13	
2		14	
3		15	
4		16	
5		17	
6		18	
7		19	
8		20	
9		21	
10		22	
11		23	
12		24	

Establishing Rewards

Remember that foods should not be labeled as good or bad or as a bribe or reward. On the other hand, remember that all types of food can fit into a balanced diet, when they are consumed wisely. High-calorie foods and beverages can add variety, pleasure, and an incentive to continue your dieting efforts. However, the best approach is to think in terms of nonfood rewards. Try one or more of the following suggestions or explore your own:

- Purchase a favorite item for every five pounds lost, such as a favorite magazine or makeup item.

- Attend a special event for every five pounds lost, such as a concert or sports activity.

- Start a new project for every five pounds lost, such as a craft or gardening.

A definite reward is a marked change in your waist circumference by noting the difference in your before-and-after pant waistline measures. Also remember your three different photos taken at the beginning, at three months, and at six months if you decided to include them. Visually witnessing the removal of those unwanted pounds by these three snapshots over time can give you a big boost in your self-confidence and in your health as well.

Female dieter image before and after showing difference between the two pant waistlines

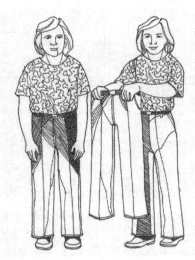

Gather Your Supportive Troops

At your meeting(s), you and your supportive partner or support team may wish to do the following:

- Share your information on the daily tracking record and weekly weight checks.

- Search the internet together for your favorite fast-food eateries for your favorite high-calorie foods and beverages and their calories and choose healthier replacements and their calories.

ENDNOTE

1   National Institutes of Health, National Heart, Lung, and Blood Institute, and North American Associates for the Study of Obesity. *The Practical Guide Identification, Evaluation, and Treatment of Overweight and Obesity in Adults.* Bethesda, MD: NIH Publication Number 02-4084, 2002.

CHAPTER
9
Planning Your Physical Activity Program

Previously, you learned that calorie intake (calories in) is only one part of the energy balance equation. The second part of this equation is energy expenditure (calories out)—that is, energy required for bodily processes to sustain life (metabolic rate) and energy required for physical activity. The ninth step on your road to better health and fitness is to develop a personal physical activity plan to make regular physical activity a lifelong practice.

The Benefits of Regular Physical Activity

An approach using both regular physical activity and a nutritionally balanced weight-loss plan is the most effective means of reducing and maintaining weight. There are a number of significant health benefits that can be acquired through regular physical activity. It is important to realize that many of these significant health benefits can be obtained through exercise *with* or *without* the loss of weight.

Weight Reduction and Maintenance

Regular physical activity can

- increase calorie expenditure, absorbing excess calories that would be used to produce excess fat, both total and at the waistline, reducing your risk for heart disease, high blood pressure, and stroke;

- minimize the loss of muscle (or lean body mass) during weight reduction, which is beneficial because lean body mass has a higher metabolic rate, burning more calories than other bodily tissues;

- include strengthening activities that involve resistance exercises that can build lean body mass; and

- be an important factor in maintaining your weight loss.

Heart and Lung Health

Regular physical activity can

- be heart-healthy because it can improve your blood pressure and blood levels of triglycerides, LDL-c, and HDL-c;

- improve the functional capacity of the heart, decreasing the risk for subsequent heart attacks; and

- promote lung health by strengthening your lung muscles, increasing the lungs' breathing capacity, especially for dieters with respiratory problems.

Normal Blood Glucose Levels

Regular physical activity can promote normal levels of blood glucose and reduce the risk of type 2 diabetes because it increases insulin-binding to cell receptors. By doing so, it increases the cell's sensitivity to insulin, resulting in a greater uptake of glucose from the blood. It reduces the risk of microvascular damage, which could result in blindness, nerve damage, or kidney failure due to excess blood glucose.

Muscle, Bone, and Joint Health

Regular physical activity can promote healthy muscles in terms of strength, tone, flexibility, and stamina as well as balance and coordination. It can also be beneficial to joints in terms of strength, stabilizing, and flexibility, especially for dieters with arthritis. By doing so, this stabilization can reduce joint pain, disability, and the need for medication. This can also apply to the reducing of knee surgery. Include strengthening activities that involve weight-bearing exercises that can promote the formation of bone, reducing the risk of osteoporosis (a disease characterized by the loss of bone mass).

Reduction of Cancer

Regular physical activity can

- reduce the risk of breast and prostate cancer, most likely due to its effect on hormone levels and

- reduce the risk of colon cancer because it stimulates a more rapid passage of stool, which often carries potential carcinogens, through the intestinal tract.

Mental Health

Regular physical activity can

- keep you healthy mentally by decreasing stress, anxiety, and depression, which could aggravate such conditions as heart disease, high blood pressure, diabetes, arthritis, or respiratory problems;

- help you become more responsible in terms of being more physically active, improving your self-esteem through increased self-discipline, confidence, and respect; and

- promote restful sleep that can provide you with the energy needed for the activities you desire and for the activities you can enjoy with your family.

Medical Advice

It is strongly recommended that you consult your physician either by phone or by visit before beginning a physical activity program, including moderate-intensity activities, as well as stretching and strengthening activities.

Based on your medical history, ask your physician to recommend one of four types of physical activity programs and what recommendations or referrals he or she would advise:

1. Unrestricted physical activity: You may be able to do any activity as long as you start slowly and build up gradually. Discuss with your doctor the activities you are interested in pursuing and what types of community or medical programs may be available to you.

2. Prescribed physical activity

3. A medically designed program of physical activity under the supervision of a trained professional, such as a physical therapist

4. No physical activity

Please note the following:

1. These recommendations need to be reviewed every six months.

2. If your health status changes within six months, notify your physician because these recommendations may be revised.

Also, it is important to note that regardless of what type of physical activity program you participate in, stop doing exercise if you experience any of these symptoms: shortness of breath, dizziness, or faintness, nausea, or chest pain. If any of these symptoms persist, call your physician immediately.

Additional Activities

The purpose of these activities related to daily routines is to keep you moving daily. Such common lifestyle activities include

- parking farther distance from entrances and getting off public transportation two blocks before your desired destination;

- climbing stairs rather than taking elevators or escalators; and

- walking or pushing a cart around perimeter aisles and inner aisles of stores.

Moderate-Intensity Activities

Moderate-intensity activities can include the following:

1. Brisk walking for thirty minutes

2. Brisk cycling for thirty minutes

3. Brisk swimming for thirty minutes

4. Any yard work, household tasks, or sports involving brisk, continuous movements for at least forty-five minutes

Sharing a physical activity with another helps you to continue this healthy practice.

Stretching Activities

Stretching activities involve simple stretches, bending, and reaching to help reduce muscle stiffness and help keep joints mobile. Strive for a slow, smooth stretch to avoid ragged or jerky movements.

The following stretching activities could be done while standing or sitting and while at home or at work. Review the arm stretches described in "Physical Relaxation Techniques" (chapter 4). Starting with your hands above your head, bend down to touch your toes. Starting with your feet on the floor, raise each leg until it is parallel to the chair or floor, and starting with your feet on the floor, raise each leg toward your chest. Try jumping jacks as well, starting with your feet together, and then jump apart and raise your hands over your head to clap at the same time. For these stretching activities, start with five stretches and gradually increase to twenty-five or thirty stretches.

In addition, most yard work, household tasks, and sports involve stretching and/or bending. Stretching activities could also include yoga. You may wish to do three to five minutes of stretching activities as warming-up and cooling-off measures before doing moderate-intensity activities.

Strengthening Activities

Strengthening activities make muscles, joints, and bones strong. Such activities require resistance exercises such as weight bearing. Two commonly practiced strengthening activities are the following:

1. Lift weights using weight-graded barbells.

2. If doing push-ups on the floor, you can use your toes or knees. Alternately, while facing a desk, chair, or wall, stand erect with your feet together and arms apart (narrow to wider) and move your head toward the desk, chair, or wall.

Other examples can include heavy yard work that requires lifting of heavy objects or daily chores that require carrying heavy items.

Practical Pointers

For moderate-intensity activities, remember to use comfortable footwear with good cushioning and support. Wear comfortable clothing (shorts, sweats, etc.) that suits the activity and weather. Wear protective gear when required, such as knee and elbow pads. These clothing and equipment recommendations are recommended for stretching and strengthening activities as well.

- Choose those activities that are enjoyable and workable for you.

- To prevent boredom, explore a variety of activities, routines, locations, and so forth. Also, periodically add new activities.

Setting Realistic Goals

Remember that physical activity should be based upon a personalized activity plan—that is, one based on personal needs and preferences. Include stretching and strengthening activities along with moderate-intensity ones.

When planning a fitness program, set goals that are achievable and sustainable. If you have been inactive, start with the less-demanding activities, such as gentle walking or swimming, and gradually add more moderate-intensity ones.

To assist you in creating your plan and adhering to it, stop at this point and give careful thought to the type of activities you want to include and the amount of time given to each activity. To help you with your planning efforts, see "Commitments to Improve My Physical Fitness" on the following pages. Also, write your responses to each section in your workbook in the appendix. An example includes a teacher who is thirty-four years of age, is married with two children, and teaches chemistry at the local high school. He plans to do the following:

- strengthening activities and the moderate-intensity activities of brisk walking and cycling in his neighborhood during the early morning

- stretching exercises in his family room and swimming in his outdoor pool after school

- weight-bearing exercises and push-ups in his family room in the evenings

- household and yard chores on Saturday

The basic purpose is to replace prolonged periods of sedentary activities with more active pursuits. In your workbook, you may wish to follow the commitment form created for this example to develop your own personal activity plan. See "Commitments to Improve My Physical Fitness."

Commitments to Improve My Physical Fitness

Section 1

In this section, list three major reasons why you want to improve your physical fitness level.

A._____

B._____

C._____

The teacher's example:

A. To help me lose weight.

B. To help me reduce my blood pressure.

C. To reduce my total LDL cholesterol levels and raise my HDL levels.

Section 2

In this section, list one or more potentially serious barriers that could block your improvement in physical fitness, and provide a solution that will help you overcome each barrier.

A._____

B. _____

C. _____

The teacher's example:

A. Lack of time: Plan ahead, schedule the time, and stick to it.

B. Lack of motivation: Recall significant health benefits of increased activity. Include in my activities my wife, children, or pet.

C. I have a busy lifestyle due to numerous family and work commitments. I will strive to simplify and better organize my time by setting priorities.

Section 3

In this section, write down the physical activity goals you wish to accomplish for each time frame.

1. First and second months: _____

2. Third and fourth months: _____

3. Fifth and sixth months: _____

The teacher's example:

First and second months:

A. Brisk walking or cycling for at least thirty minutes, five days weekly, and household chores or yard work for at least forty-five minutes, one day weekly

B. Simple stretching exercises or swimming for ten minutes at least two days weekly

C. Lifting weights and doing push-ups for ten minutes at least two days weekly

Third and fourth months:

A. Brisk walking or cycling for at least forty-five minutes, six days weekly, and houschold chores or yard work for at least forty-five minutes one day weekly

B. Simple stretching exercises or swimming for fifteen minutes at least two days weekly

C. Lifting weights and doing push-ups for fifteen minutes at least two days weekly

Fifth and sixth months:

A. Brisk walking or cycling for at least sixty minutes daily and household chores or yard work for at least forty-five minutes one day weekly

B. Simple stretching exercises or swimming for twenty minutes at least two days weekly

C. Lifting weights and doing push-ups for twenty minutes at least two days weekly

Recording Your Physical Fitness Progress

Now, let us consider how you can record the amount of each physical activity you have done.

Keeping a Log of Activities

The simplest way to record in your workbook are the amounts of your activities in a weekly log. From this log, you will be able to see your weekly pattern of activity, as well as identifying any problematic areas, such as extended periods of inactivity.

You will be able to answer such important questions as: How much time is spent on sedentary activities versus moderate-intensity activities? How active you are on weekdays versus weekend days (or on days you work versus days spent off work)? Which activities would you like to increase and to decrease, according to your physician's advice? For an example of this log format, see "The Teacher's Weekly Log of Physical Activities."

The Teacher's Weekly Log of Physical Activities

Sixth Month: June 1–7, 2018
Monday
Brisk walking, sixty minutes
Stretching activities, twenty minutes

Tuesday
Brisk cycling, sixty minutes
Lifting weights/push-ups (strengthening), twenty minutes

Wednesday
Brisk walking, sixty minutes
Swimming (stretching), twenty minutes

Thursday
Brisk cycling, sixty minutes
Lifting weights/pushups (strengthening), twenty minutes

Friday
Brisk walking, sixty minutes

Saturday
Brisk cycling, sixty minutes
Yard work, forty-five minutes

Sunday
Brisk cycling, sixty minutes

Summary: Brisk walking or cycling for sixty minutes for seven days; stretching exercises or swimming for twenty minutes for two days; lifting weights/pushups (strengthening) for twenty minutes for two days; and household chores or yardwork for forty five minutes for one day weekly.

Monitoring Your Walking Experience

As an alternative to logging your walking activities in minutes, determine the number of steps you have taken. Use a pedometer (or an activity tracker). Practical advice regarding pedometers is as follows:

- Gradually increase your steps by two hundred steps each week or whatever time frame you feel comfortable with until you reach at least two thousand steps in thirty minutes.

- Keep a daily log of your activities (date and number of steps).

- As with other fitness equipment, it is best to investigate the internet resources because they have a wider range of pedometer (or activity tracker) options and prices.

Rewarding Your Physical Fitness Efforts

During this initial six-month period of your fitness program, remember to reward yourself periodically as you progress toward meeting your fitness goals. See the information about rewards in chapter 8.

Making Fitness a Family Affair

If you become active, your children will become as well. Have family members plan a family-centered activity at least once or twice monthly (or as often as possible), such as walking together, biking, hiking, or swimming.

Family-centered activities promote health as well as helping family members communicate with each other.

Gather Your Supportive Troops

At your meeting(s), share your fitness plan with your supportive partner or support team:

- Enlist the aid of other supportive individuals by making your physical activity program a family affair or by asking friends, neighbors, or coworkers to participate in the activities.

- Being with a supportive person or group is very important in maintaining walking as a regular exercise.

- You may also wish to share your ideas about keeping a log of your physical activities.

CHAPTER
10 Weight Maintenance

Weight maintenance occurs when there is a balance between your energy intake (calories in) and your energy expenditure (calories out). In addition to using weekly weight checks to track weight loss, such weekly checks can help you maintain weight by decreasing intake or increasing activity level when a slight weight gain is first observed.

Why is weight maintenance important? Weight cycling and yo-yo dieting are terms that refer to repeated episodes of weight loss and weight regain. Such weight-loss and regain episodes not only can cause emotional stress and continued discouragement but can be harmful physically as well. Positive changes in your weight, health (mental and physical), diet, eating practices, and physical activity can be a powerful reward for the shedding of those unhealthy pounds and keeping them off and most of all, achieving a better quality of life.

It is difficult to lose weight, but a more challenging task is to maintain this weight loss. It is very important to continue to practice those healthy behaviors you have learned, while guarding against returning to those old, unhealthy ones. The goal of this chapter is to provide you with practical advice that will help you retain the weight you have lost.

The tenth step on your road to better health and fitness is tallying your improvements during weight loss and selecting a weight-maintenance plan and making commitments (or goals) for further improvement.

Summary of the Benefits of Your Weight-Loss Efforts

The purpose of this guide is to provide you with the evaluation tools and professional advice to promote a gradual loss of weight and small, incremental changes in lifestyle practices that are required to sustain this weight loss over time. Popular, quick-fix diets fail to promote such permanent lifestyle behavior changes. Over the past six months, you have worked hard at meeting your commitments to improve your weight, health, dietary intake, eating practices, and physical activity levels. Additionally, you have striven to reduce the amount of stress in your life and improve your psychological well-being for these commitments to be realized. Now take a few minutes to study the following simplified, schematic diagram that summarizes these efforts. This diagram shows how self-improvement through positive lifestyle changes can result in better health. Note the reinforcing nature of these positive changes.

Positive Lifestyle Changes for Better Health

If you reduce your stress level and make positive changes in your psychological factors (such as body image), including improved dietary intake, eating practices, and physical activity, improved BMI, waist circumference, and weight, improved metabolic parameters as (blood pressure), and reduced risk for the chronic diseases, all of these improvements from dietary intake to reduced risk for disease reinforces your reduced stress level and positive psychological factors.

Evaluating Your Weight-Loss Efforts

For this evaluation, return to your workbook in the appendix and provide the information for chapters 1–4 and 6–7 for six months. To determine improvement, compare your results at the beginning of your weight-loss efforts with those at six months. As you read through the following questions in each chapter, write down your answers in your workbook. Circle in green those practices that no longer require improvement; in yellow, those in which some improvement has been made; and in red, those practices where no improvement was made.

Chapter 1: To improve my weight.

- How much weight did you lose? _____ pounds.

- How much did your BMI decrease? From _____ to _____.

- Did your BMI weight status improve? Status initially _____ to status at six months _____.

- How much did your waist circumference decrease? _____ inches.

- Did your waist circumference change from high risk to low risk for disease? Yes or no.

Chapter 2: To improve my health.

Did you improve the following?

- Blood pressure? Some decrease or from abnormal to borderline or borderline to normal or abnormal to normal or no improvement.

- Blood glucose levels? Some decrease or from abnormal to borderline or borderline to normal or abnormal to normal or no improvement.

- Blood LDL-c levels? Some decrease or from abnormal to borderline or borderline to normal or abnormal to normal or no improvement.

- Blood HDL-c levels? Some increase or from abnormal to normal or no improvement.

- Blood triglyceride levels? Some decrease or from abnormal to borderline or borderline to normal or abnormal to normal or no improvement.

Chapter 3: To prepare myself mentally.

Did you improve the following?

- Self-concept rating? 1 to 2, 2 to 3, 3 to 4, 4 to 5, or 5 to 6 or other (3 to 5) or no improvement

- Body image rating? 1 to 2, 2 to 3, 3 to 4, 4 to 5, or 5 to 6 or other (2 to 4) or no improvement

- Self-esteem rating? 1 to 2, 2 to 3, 3 to 4, 4 to 5, or 5 to 6 or other (2 to 4) or no improvement

Chapter 4: To reduce my stress level.

- Did you reduce your stress level based on the five-point scale? From 5 to 4, 4 to 3, 3 to 2, 2 to 1, or other (4 to 2) or no improvement.

Chapter 5: To learn basic nutrition facts and information about nutrition labeling.

- Did you find any cereals that had high iron and fiber content that you purchased and liked? Yes or no?

- Did you find any whole-grain products that had a high fiber content that you purchased and liked? Yes or no?

- Did you find any fat-free or lower-fat products that you purchased and liked? Yes or no?

Chapter 6: To improve my dietary intake.

In a typical week, how many days did you meet the recommendation? See "Weekly Tracking Record of Food Groups."

- At least three servings of a calcium-rich source daily? 0 to 1, 1 to 2, 2 to 3, 3 to 4, 4 to 5, 5 to 6, or 6 to 7 days or other (4 to 6) or no improvement.

- At least five servings of fruits and vegetables daily? 0 to 1, 1 to 2, 2 to 3, 3 to 4, 4 to 5, 5 to 6, or 6 to 7 days or other (2 to 4) or no improvement.

- Within the five servings, at least one serving of a vitamin A–rich fruit or vegetable daily (minimum three days)? 0 to 1, 1 to 2, 2 to 3, 3 to 4, 4 to 5, 5 to 6, or 6 to 7 days or other (1 to 3) or no improvement.

- Within the five servings, at least one serving of a vitamin C–rich fruit or vegetable daily? 0 to 1, 1 to 2, 2 to 3, 3 to 4, 4 to 5, 5 to 6, or 6 to 7 days or other (5 to 7) or no improvement.

- At least three servings of whole-grain products daily? 0 to 1, 1 to 2, 2 to 3, 3 to 4, 4 to 5, 5 to 6, or 6 to 7 days or other (3 to 5) or no improvement.

- No more than one alcoholic beverage daily for men and women? From more than one drink daily to one drink daily or no improvement. 0 to 1, 1 to 2, 2 to 3, 3 to 4, 4 to 5, 5 to 6, or 6 to 7 days or other (2 to 4) or no improvement

Chapter 7: To improve my eating practices.

Write down your percentage for each of the following eating practices at the beginning of your weight-loss efforts. For at least 90 percent of your meals and snacks weekly, did you meet this recommendation? Write down yes or no. Then write down your percentage at six months.

- Eat regular meals and snacks? Percent = () yes or no to percent = () at six months yes or no or no improvement

- Respond to your feelings of being hungry or being full to start and stop eating? Percent = () yes or no to percent = () at six months yes or no or no improvement

- Eat recommended portion (or serving) sizes? Percent = () yes or no to percent = () at six months yes or no or no improvement

How many days of the week did you meet the recommendation?

- Have family meals? 0 to 1, 1 to 2, 2 to 3, 3 to 4, or 5 days or more weekly or other (2 to 4) or no improvement?

- Slow your pace of eating so that major meals each day last between twenty to thirty minutes? 0 to 1, 1 to 2, 2 to 3, 3 to 4, 4 to 5, 5 to 6, or 7 days or other (4 to 6) or no improvement.

- A high-calorie food at a meal or snack? 7 to 6, 6 to 5, 5 to 4, or 3 days, or less weekly or other (6 to 4) or no improvement? If you have two or more servings of such foods daily, estimate the number of days you do so.

- Drink a high-calorie beverage at a meal or snack daily? More than one beverage daily to only one beverage daily or no improvement? If you have two or more servings of a high-calorie beverage daily, estimate the number of days you do so. Align the days.

- Eat in rooms other than the kitchen or dining area while doing other activities? 7 to 6, 6 to 5, 5 to 4, or 3 days or less or other (7 to 5), or no improvement. If you do this practice more than once daily, estimate the number of days you do so. Align the days.

- Eat a meal or snack at a restaurant or fast-food establishment? 7 to 6, 6 to 5, 5 to 4, 4 to 3, or 2 days or less weekly or other (5 to 3) or no improvement. If you do this practice more than once daily, estimate the number of days you do so. Align the days.

- Emotionally overeat? 7 to 6, 6 to 5, 5 to 4, 4 to 3, 3 to 2, 2 to 1, 1 to 0 days, or other (4 to 2) or no improvement. If you do this practice more than once daily, estimate the number of days you do so. Align the days.

Chapter 8: To follow my weight-loss plan.

- Did you follow your weight-loss plan at least 90 percent of the time? Yes or no? To determine this, see "Weekly Tracking Record of Food Groups" and divide the number of days you followed your plan by the number of days recorded and then multiply by 100. Your percent _____.

- Did you follow your weight-loss plan at least 90 percent of the time on weekend days? Yes or no? To determine this, see "Weekly Tracking Record of Food Groups" and divide the number of weekend days you followed your plan by the number of weekend days recorded and then multiply by 100. Your percent _____.

Chapter 9: To follow my physical activity plan.

- Did you follow your physical activity plan at least 90 percent of the time? Yes or no? To determine this, see your log of physical activity in your workbook. Divide the number of weeks you followed your plan by the number of weekly logs recorded and multiply by 100. Your percent _____.

If you have improved or partly improved some of the above practices in your evaluation, congratulations! If all of your medical parameters are within the normal range, like blood pressure, this is a milestone on your road to better health and fitness.

Determining Your Weight-Maintenance Plan

For your weight-maintenance plan, start with your intake that you determined by your three-day log of intake, specifically, the number of servings for each of the food groups. Because you have lost weight, you require fewer calories to move your lighter body. Because of this, you will need to adjust the number of servings of the different food groups to lower your calorie intake. If you have lost twenty to twenty-five pounds, decrease your intake by two servings from the grain group and one serving from the fat group; twenty-six to thirty pounds, decrease your intake by two servings from the grain group and two servings from the fat group; thirty-one to thirty-five pounds, decrease your intake by two servings from the grain group, two servings from the fat group, and one ounce of lean meat; thirty-six to forty pounds, decrease your intake by two servings from the grain group, two servings from the fat group, and two ounces of lean meat; forty-one to forty-five pounds, decrease your intake by three servings from the grain group, two servings from the fat group, and one ounce of lean meat; and forty-six to fifty pounds, decrease your intake by three servings from the grain group, two servings from the fat group, and two ounces of lean meat. This plan will become your weight-maintenance plan.

It is very important to continue your physical activity plan during weight maintenance. In addition to the physical activity recommendations in chapter 8, work hard to avoid lengthy periods of inactivity—for example, working on your computer or watching television for entertainment and talking or texting on your phone. Keep moving!

After a six-month weight-maintenance period, if you wish to reduce your weight further, follow the recommendations for selecting a weight-loss plan in chapter 8.

You may wish to review the "Serving Sizes for the Weight-Loss Plans," "Selections and Preparation Tips," "Special Considerations," "Recommended Eating Practices to Improve While Reducing Your

Weight," "Recommended Physical Activity While Reducing Your Weight," "Planning Healthy Meals and Snacks," and "Establishing Rewards" in chapter 8, for they also apply to your weight-maintenance plan. Also, use the dietary tracking form and weekly weight check form, and keep a log of your physical activity.

Making Commitments Related to Healthy Practices for the Weight-Maintenance Period and for the Future

I would advise the following concerning commitments involving lifestyle practices. Such lifestyle practices include your level of stress, psychological factors, dietary intake, eating practices, and physical activity level:

- Continue those practices (circled in green) that have met the recommendation for that practice and no longer require improvement.

- Focus on those practices (circled in yellow) that require additional improvement and those practices (circled in red) where no improvement was made.

- Whether you have a continued weight maintenance or decide to reduce your weight further, every six months, make a commitment to improve one or two of those practices circled in yellow or red for months one and two, three and four, and five and six months.

Gather Your Supportive Troops

At your meeting(s), you and your supportive partner or support team may share the results of your evaluation and help each other by brainstorming ideas for commitments during weight maintenance and for the future.

Good luck with your weight-loss and weight-maintenance efforts! Keep in mind that if you need to discontinue your weight-loss or weight-maintenance efforts for any reason, you can always return to this book and restart your efforts.

Appendix

Workbook of My Progress

I would advise that you apply the colors of a traffic light, using colored pencils, to identify the positive changes observed in your results from the different chapters by doing the following: circle in green those results that do not need improvement; yellow for those results where some improvement has been made; and those in red needing improvement. This color scheme is a quick and colorful way to show your positive changes.

Chapter 1: Step 1: To evaluate my weight.

For the following information, see the weight status and waist circumference risk for disease classifications in chapter 1. For weight status, circle in red (the three types of obesity), in yellow (overweight), and in green (normal). For waist circumference risk for disease, circle in red (high) and in green (low). Do the following.

1. Write down your height.

2. Write down the following weight-related information at the beginning, at three months, and at six months during your weight-loss efforts.

    A. Write down your weight (pounds) (e.g., 168)

    B. Your BMI (weight status) (e.g., twenty-eight, overweight)

    C. Your waist circumference (inches) (risk for disease) (e.g., thirty-six, high)

Chapter 2: Step 2: To evaluate my health.

Medical Parameters

Circle in red (abnormal), in yellow (borderline) (if needed), and in green (normal):

1. Write down your blood pressure readings (mm/hg) at the beginning, at three months, and at six months (e.g., 142/94, abnormal).

2. Write down the following blood-related risk factors at the beginning, three months (if needed), and six months.

    A. Glucose (mg/dl) (e.g., 99, normal)

    B. LDL-c levels (mg/dl)

    C. HDL-c levels (mg/dl)

    D. Triglyceride levels (mg/dl)

Medications

Write down the medication(s) prescribed by your physician, including its name, purpose, and total daily dosage at the beginning, at three months, and at six months. If there are any increases in dosage, circle in red; if the dosage remains the same, circle in yellow; and if there are any decreases in dosages, circle in green.

Chapter 3: Step 3: Adopt positive thoughts about myself and my weight.

Record the following at the beginning of your weight-loss efforts and at six months. Write down the following:

1. Self-Concept: Your answers to the ten questions (section 1), for example, loving, AG. Circle in red, those answers that are marked

DG; in yellow, those marked as UN; and in green, those marked as AG.

2. Body Image: Your answers to the five questions (section 2), for example, physical appearance, AG. Circle in red those answers that are marked as AG; in yellow, those marked as UN; and in green, those marked as DG.

3. Self-Esteem: Your answers to the five questions (section 3), for example, self-acceptance, AG. Circle in red those answers that are marked as DG; in yellow, those marked as UN; and in green, those marked as AG.

Record the following at the beginning of your weight-loss efforts and at six months. Write down your ratings of the three concepts based on the six-point scale. Circle in red those ratings of 1 or 2; in yellow, those ratings of 3 or 4; and in green, those ratings of 5 or 6:

A. Your self-concept (e.g., 4)

B. Body image (e.g., 3)

C. Self-esteem (e.g., 3)

Chapter 4: Step 4: To reduce stress.

Record the following at the beginning of your weight-loss efforts and at six months.

1. Write down how you rate your stress level on the following five-point scale: 1, slightly stressed; 2, somewhat stressed; 3, fairly stressed; 4, moderately stressed; and 5, very stressed, at the beginning of your weight loss efforts and at six months. For example, 5 is very stressed at the beginning and 3 is fairly stressed at six months. Circle in red the ratings of moderately and very stressful; in yellow, the ratings of somewhat and fairly stressful; and in green, the rating of slightly stressful.

2. Write down your three major sources of stress and the mental and/or relaxation techniques that you have chosen to reduce such stress.

3. At six months, if your stress level is not reduced to "slightly stressed," continue with the same three stress areas, but try different relaxation techniques that may be more effective. If your stress level is reduced to "slightly stressed," continue with the same sources of stress and techniques, but you may wish to add one or two other sources and techniques to reduce stress in these areas.

Chapter 5: Step 5: To learn basic nutritional information and facts about labeling.

Before beginning your weight-loss efforts, survey your favorite grocery stores for the following products. Include those products that you are most likely to purchase. I would suggest that you take with you a small spiral notebook to write down new products:

1. Compare cereals: Write down the store, the product (plus brand name), calories per serving, serving size, percent of iron, and grams of fiber for each product.

2. Discover whole-grain products. Write down the store, the product (plus brand name), calories per serving, serving size, and grams of fiber for whole-grain breads, buns, rolls, pastas, wild rice, crackers, chips, and snack products.

3. Explore lower-fat products: Write down the store, the product (plus brand name), calories per serving, serving size, and grams of fat for the following products. Dieters often shy away from such products, questioning their acceptability. I have tried many lower-fat products and have found them to be quite acceptable, flavorful, and satisfying.

Fat-Free or Lower-Fat Dairy Products

1. Fat-free (skim) and low-fat (1 percent) milk

2. 2 percent milk

3. Fat-free or lower-fat yogurts (plain or flavored)

4. Fat-free frozen yogurts

5. Fat-free ice creams

Meat and Alternatives

1. Lean meat and hamburger with the lowest percent of fat or alternative:

    A. Lower-fat cottage cheese

    B. Lower-fat cheeses

    C. Lower-fat processed sandwich meats

    D. Lower-fat hot dogs and sausage

    E. Tuna (reduced-fat, water-packed, or drained of oil)

Grain Products

1. Bread (reduced calories)

2. Lower-fat popcorn products

3. Lower-fat snack chips (potato or tortilla)

Sweets and Desserts

1. Sugar-free Jell-O

2. Sugar-free puddings (made with lower-fat milk)

Fats

1. Fat-free or lower-fat salad dressings and mayonnaise

2. Fat-free or lower-fat cream cheese and sour cream

3. Other low-fat foods

Combination Foods

1. Frozen meals less than 350 calories

2. 2 other products (you may think of or discover these)

Chapter 6: Step 6: To improve my dietary intake.

Record your results before beginning your weight-loss efforts and at six months.

Write down the number of days you met the recommendations for the sources of calcium, fruits and vegetables in general, fruits and vegetables high in vitamins A and C, whole-grain products, and alcohol intake. Behind the number of days, answer yes if you met the recommendation for all seven days or no, if you did not. For example, sources of calcium for five days, no. Circle in green your answers of yes or in red, your answers of no.

Chapter 7: Step 7: To improve my eating practices.

Record the following information at the beginning of your weight-loss efforts and at six months.

Write down the three eating practices with the phrase 90 percent (on a weekly basis). Answer yes or no to the 90 percent recommendation. If you do not, write down the percentage you are doing presently.

Circle in green your answers yes, and in red, your answers no. For example: 90 percent, your percent, 90 percent (six months); eat regular meals and snacks no, 60, yes.

For the remaining eating practices, write down the number of days you met the specific recommendation. Did it match the total number of days recommended? Yes or no? For example, family meals (three days). No, five days recommended. Circle in green your answers yes and in red, your answers no.

Chapter 8: Step 8: To select a realistic weight-loss plan.

1. Keep your three-day log here and the results of the five subsequent steps related to it.

2. Write down the number of servings for each of the food groups that make up your weight-loss plan.

3. Write down the results of the internet search: the name of the fast-food establishment, your favorite high-calorie foods and beverages and their calories, and your healthier replacements and their calories.

4. Write down your answers of yes or no to the questions about how your weekend days differ from your weekdays in terms of intake. For example, more calories, yes, circle in red your answers in yes and in green your answers of no.

Chapter 9: Step 9: To develop a personal physical activity plan.

1. Write down your responses to the three sections of "Commitments to Improve My Physical Fitness."

2. Keep an ongoing log of your physical activities, including the date, the activity, and the amount of time spent on the activity. For walking, you may also record it as steps determined by a

pedometer or activity tracker. Place a green X by those weeks you followed your physical activity plan.

Chapter 10: Step 10: Tally your improvements during weight loss and select a weight-maintenance plan:

1. Write down the number of servings for each of the food groups that make up your weight-maintenance diet.

2. Every six months, write down the one or two practices that you wish to improve during months one and two, three and four, and five and six.

3. As you read through the questions related to each chapter presented shortly, write down your answers from the choices given. To determine improvement, compare your results at the beginning of your weight-loss efforts with those at six months. Circle in green those practices that no longer require improvement; in yellow, those where some improvement has been made; and in red, areas where improvement is necessary.

Chapter 1: To improve my weight.

- How much weight did you lose?

- How much did your BMI decrease?

- Did your BMI weight status improve?

- How much did your waist circumference decrease?

- Did your waist circumference change from high risk to low risk for disease?

Chapter 2: To improve my health.

Did you improve your blood pressure? Consider the following:

- blood glucose levels

- blood LDL-c levels

- blood HDL-c levels

- blood triglyceride levels

Chapter 3: To prepare myself mentally.

Did you improve these areas:

- self-concept rating

- body image rating

- self-esteem rating

Chapter 4: To reduce my stress level.

- Did you reduce your stress level based on the five-point scale?

Chapter 5: To learn basic nutrition facts and information about nutrition labeling.

- Did you find any cereals that had high iron and fiber contents that you purchased and liked?

- Did you find any whole-grain products that had a high fiber content that you purchased and liked?

- Did you find any fat-free or lower-fat products that you purchased and liked?

Chapter 6: To improve my dietary intake.

In a typical week, how many days did you consume the following:

- at least three servings of a calcium-rich source daily

- at least five servings of fruits and vegetables daily

- within the five servings, at least one serving of a vitamin A–rich fruit or vegetables daily (minimum three days)

- within the five servings, at least one serving of a vitamin C–rich fruit or vegetables daily

- at least three servings of whole-grain products daily

- no more than one alcoholic beverage daily for men and women

Chapter 7: To improve my eating practices.

For at least 90 percent of your meals and snacks weekly, did you meet this recommendation? If your answer is no, write down the percentage you did so.

- ate regular meals and snacks

- responded to your feelings of being hungry or being full to start and stop eating

- ate recommended portion (or serving) sizes

- days of per week that you met the recommendation

- had family meals

- slowed your pace of eating

- ate high-calorie food at a meal or snack (If you have two or more servings of such foods daily, estimate the number of days you do so. Align the days.)

- drank a high-calorie beverage at a meal or a snack daily (If you have two or more servings of a high-calorie beverage daily, estimate the number of days you do so. Align the days.)

- ate in rooms other than the kitchen or dining area while doing other activities (If you do this practice more than once daily, estimate the number of days you do so. Align the days.)

- ate a meal or snack at a restaurant or fast-food establishment (If you do this practice more than once daily, estimate the number of days you do so. Align the days.)

- emotionally overate (If you do this practice more than once daily, estimate the number of days you do so. Align the days.)

Chapter 8: To follow my weight-loss plan.

- Did you follow your weight-loss plan at least 90 percent of the time?

- Did you follow your weight-loss plan at least 90 percent of the time on weekend days?

Chapter 9: To follow my physical activity plan.

- Did you follow your physical activity plan at least 90 percent of the time?

Index

Printed in the United States
By Bookmasters